WITHDRAWN

Carnegie Mellon

Strategic Issues and Challenges in Health Management

Strategic Issues and Challenges in Health Management

Edited by

K.V. Ramani
Dileep Mavalankar
Dipti Govil

Centre for Management of Health Services (CMHS)
Indian Institute of Management, Ahmedabad

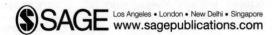

Los Angeles • London • New Delhi • Singapore
www.sagepublications.com

Copyright © K.V. Ramani, Dileep Mavalankar and Dipti Govil, 2008

First published in 2008 by

SAGE Publications India Pvt Ltd
B 1/I-1 Mohan Cooperative Industrial Area
Mathura Road, New Delhi 110 044, India
www.sagepub.in

SAGE Publications Inc
2455 Teller Road
Thousand Oaks, California 91320, USA

SAGE Publications Ltd
1 Oliver's Yard, 55 City Road
London EC1Y 1SP, United Kingdom

SAGE Publications Asia-Pacific Pte Ltd
33 Pekin Street
#02-01 Far East Square
Singapore 048763

and

Centre for Management of Health Services (CMHS)
Indian Institute of Management
Vastrapur, Ahmedabad 308 051, India

Published by Vivek Mehra for SAGE Publications India Pvt Ltd, typeset in 10.5/12.5pt Charter BT by Star Compugraphics Private Limited, Delhi and printed at Chaman Enterprises, New Delhi.

Library of Congress Cataloging-in-Publication Data

Strategic issues and challenges in health management/edited by K.V. Ramani,
    Dileep Mavalankar, and Dipti Govil.
       p. cm.
    Includes bibliographical references and index.
    1. Health care reform—India.   2. Medical policy—India.   3. Health planning—
India. I. Ramani, K.V. II. Mavalankar, Dileep. III. Govil, Dipti. [DNLM:
1. Delivery of Health Care—organization & administration—India. 2. Health
Planning—India. 3. Health Policy—India. 4. Public Health Practice—India. 5.
Socioeconomic Factors—India. WA 84 JI4 S898 2008]

RA395.I5S77   362.1'04250954—dc22   2008   2008016122

ISBN: 978-0-7619-3654-1 (HB)   978-81-7829-820-7 (India-HB)

The SAGE Team: Sugata Ghosh, Anushree Tiwari, Mathew P.J. and
                    Trinankur Banerjee

Contents

List of Tables

List of Figures

List of Maps

List of Maps

Introduction

Health and socio-economic developments are so closely intertwined that it is impossible to achieve one without the other. While economic development in India has been gaining momentum over the last decade, our health system is at crossroads today. Even though government initiatives in public health have recorded some noteworthy successes over time, the Indian health system is ranked 118 among 191 WHO member countries on overall health performance. Building health systems that are responsive to community needs, particularly for the poor, requires politically difficult and administratively demanding choices. Health is a priority goal in its own right, as well as a central input to economic development and poverty reduction. The health sector is complex with multiple goals, multiple products and different beneficiaries. India is well placed now to develop a uniquely Indian set of health sector reforms to enable the health system in meeting the increasing expectations of its users and staff. There are many managerial challenges: to ensure availability, access, affordability and equity in delivering health services to meet the community needs efficiently and effectively.

The contributed chapters in this book are organised into 10 thematic areas, which cover important strategic issues in health care in India. We begin with health system planning and development. Planning and development are very important issues in low resource settings where health and socio-economic development are closely linked. Health services are seen as an investment in reducing the burden of disease and enhancing development. The current developments in globalisation and changes in technology pose new challenges and require long term vision to address some health development challenges like equity, access, cost effectiveness etc. Health planning and development is closely linked to the way the health sector is financed. Financing can be a major tool of increasing equity in health care—especially in a mixed health care system where both public and private providers are present. Financing mechanisms can also lead to better accountability of the public system. Public-Private Partnership (PPP) is an area of great interest and debate in health systems in India. It is believed that through PPP the health system can achieve better utilisation of resources, higher efficiency and easier access. Examples of PPP in the TB control programme in India provide such hope. Even in Sri Lanka, where it is a largely public service dominated system, PPP holds hope for better health services.

Of late, governance issues are emerging as major barriers to development, including health development. Many strategic issues like what type of health care to offer, where to locate health facilities and how to ensure the delivery of best possible care without raising unnecessary barriers to care are closely linked to the governance structure of the health system. Governance issues arise in private as well as public sector health care institutions. Capacity development of the health system needs leadership and good management. The quality of care is highly dependent on the capacity of the staff and systems; the Aravind Eye Care System in India has developed the capacity of its paramedical staff to provide high quality care at low cost on a massive scale.

National health programmes are the backbone of public health in India. The way national health programmes are structured and implemented needs a lot of thought and strategic management as the country is very diverse with uneven capacities and varying needs. The National Rural Health Mission is trying to revamp the health system and make it more client oriented and cost effective. The Millennium Development Goals (MDG) have provided a global framework for directing development programmes globally. The key health-related MDGs focus on maternal and child health, infectious diseases including HIV/AIDS, TB and malaria. The MDGs also provide inter-sectoral perspective on poverty reduction where health is a part of it. For long, health planners have focussed on supply of services rather than demand from the community and linkages with the community. The experiences of some states in India show that community-based volunteers for health are effective in changing community perspective and improving health.

Urban health was neglected for a long time by the national health planners in India. It was left to local municipal authorities who have very little capacity and interest in preventive and public health. But of late several efforts have been made to highlight the importance of urban health as India is rapidly becoming an urbanised country. India, like many other developing countries, is facing demographic and epidemiological (disease) transitions. Both communicable and non-communicable diseases are rising rapidly due to increased longevity and unplanned growth in urban India. The strategic thrust in health development must focus on this transition of disease pattern. This calls for capable and well-trained human resources, as well as a good management planning and monitoring system.

Summaries of papers under each theme

Health systems planning and development

Jeffrey D. Sachs, in his remarks on 'Scaling up Health in Low Income Settings', discusses certain critical issues related to health and economic development. Health, in many ways, is a major spur to overall economic development. For example, reduction in fertility increases economic status and better health leads to greater productivity. However, good health largely depends on the health system and the general environment, both social and infrastructural, in which people live. India suffers from the dual disease burden of traditional infections and modern lifestyle diseases. The public health system in India has an organised hierarchy from the village to the union level. However, a dreadful gap can be observed between the theory on paper and the actual practice. Therefore, the people at all income levels avoid the state-run system and avail the services from private providers. Finance management, implementation of close-to-client system and recruitment of village health workers are three important issues for improving the Indian public health system. These remarks are based on the report of the Commission on Macroeconomics and Health, which he chaired.

Andrew Green in his chapter 'Health Systems: A 2020 Vision' addresses the issues related to the future challenges facing health systems with respect to contextual changes, globalisation, governance, economic and political shifts, natural and artificial crisis, urbanisation, environmental degradation, technology, health care and consumer expectation at both national and international levels. The likely health needs in 2020 indicate concerns for the burden of 15 leading non-communicable diseases. Developing health systems should also respond to general expansion of services, types of health care offered, ownership and roles of health agencies, types of health professionals, economic implications, community engagement models, management issues and multi-sectoral challenges. Above all, any health system should pursue equity of health, and thereby strengthen global policy mechanisms.

Health care financing

On the subject of equity in health financing, G. N. V. Ramana indicates that programmes and facilities must be targeted and made more accessible to the poor so as to eliminate the inequity and make services pro-poor, especially in the private sector. Under the framework of World Development Report 2004, he suggests that the best way to make services work for the poor is by strengthening direct accountability mechanisms while empowering clients with information, and their involvement in co-producing services or demand-side financing. It is possible to achieve some of these objectives through public-private participation. Some good examples of accountability mechanisms can be found in education (scholarships), nutrition supplement (free basic health care package), etc. which directly reach the needy population through effective and transparent target mechanisms.

Public-Private Partnership

Meenakshi Datta Ghosh, in her chapter 'Public-Private Partnerships in Health Care' addresses the opportunities for potential advantages and disadvantages of PPP. In 2004, eight median districts (CMIE index 1991) were evaluated from the states of West Bengal, Maharashtra, Andhra Pradesh, Bihar, Uttar Pradesh, Madhya Pradesh and Rajasthan. The ratio of public-private facilities was found to be 60:40 in rural areas and 10:90 in urban areas, indicating a need to revise the models for the relocation of primary health care facilities. PPP design at primary health care levels should be based on a range of services rather than only on one-time activities. To achieve this, it is necessary to perform detailed micro-planning of facilities, especially at the primary level. Some of the anticipated outcomes of a PPP are cost effectiveness, higher productivity, and accelerated delivery of goods resulting from a shared use of available resources.

Muraleedharan and his colleagues in their chapter 'Private-Public Participation in the Control of Tuberculosis...', describe the learning from a primary study they conducted to understand policy challenges in strengthening PPP in the implementation of Revised National Tuberculosis Control Programme (RNTCP). Their study covers 400 key informants and 118 TB patients in Tamil Nadu and Kerala. The RNTCP has a specific scheme to involve private practitioners and Non-Governmental Organisations (NGOs) in Directly Observed Treatment (DOT) implementation throughout the country. Their study brings out three critical reasons for adopting PPP, namely, cost-effectiveness, access to care and sharing financial burden. Issues related to grant-in-aid and incentives, field staff recruitment and training, and regular inspection need special attention. Future success of the PPP strategy in the implementation of RNTCP depends, to a great extent, on careful nurturing of NGOs and community volunteers committed to promoting public health.

Sri Lanka has a better-managed primary and secondary health care service delivery system. It is one of the most progressive and unique models of public-private partnership, from which other developing countries can learn. More than 50 per cent of Sri Lanka's national health expenditure comes from private sources since the last two decades. While talking about the experience of public-private partnership in Sri Lanka, Aruna Rabel mentions the problems and underlying challenges during the initial stages of establishing PPP such as inefficient utilisation of available resources, unnecessary investment by both sectors, increased cost of health care, obstacles to quality assurance, inadequately planned health care delivery, training of health care personnel and health care planning. Over a period of time, Sri Lanka's approach in implementing a PPP model for health care has expanded the reach of its health network, benefiting health sector professionals as well as its people.

Governance in health

S. R. Rao, in his chapter 'Governance in Health Systems', emphasises the need for restructuring the health services. Public-Private Partnership could aid in meeting the health care demands. Training of health volunteers, effective referral systems and affordable services are some of the necessary elements to overcome poor health conditions. Low-cost curative centres with modern equipments, organised logistics, and financial and technical support to voluntary health agencies will also bring positive results. Services devoted to special segments of the society (mentally retarded, deaf, dumb, blind, etc.), including elderly populations, are other issues that need to be addressed. Above all, an effective health information system is required for the planning, decision-making, forecasting, reviewing and monitoring of the programmes.

H. Sudarshan in his chapter 'Good Governance in Health Services' states that India is ranked 88 out of 158 countries on Transparency International's corruption index. Transparency International India, in its empirical survey on corruption, states that Bihar is the most corrupt state and Kerala is the least. According to Transparency International, corruption in health services is the second major issue of concern. Logistics, doctors and paramedical staff, civil work, administration and medical education are the major source of corruption in health sector. Private hospitals are not different from the public sector with regard to corruption. Sudarshan indicates that capacity building in health and hospital management, leadership, decision-making and problem-solving have somewhat addressed the issue of corruption. Effective management and supervision, e-governance for transparency and accountability, training in health management, hospital committees, citizen's charter, report card system, etc., are other avenues available to minimise corruption in health systems.

Capacity development

Joe Curian discusses leadership qualities in his chapter 'Strategic Leadership and Health Care Delivery'. He states that the qualities needed in a leader may not be different in the hospital industry as compared to other industries. A typical function of a strategic leader involves perception of the environment. A leader shall not only cover the emerging opportunities in the market place from the customers' point of view (society at large) but also other businesses, which will help in planning for new products/services. A strategic leader must keep perceiving the changes around, conceiving the changes and finally, delivering the changes. A leader may not have all the answers but should have all the right questions. He must have a high degree of tolerance and patience to listen to his juniors and other professionals. With growing opportunities for the health care business, innovation and creativity will become very crucial for successful leaders. It can be said that true leadership converts ordinary performers into heroes who are the link between the past and the future.

The United Nations defines Capacity Development as a process that 'focuses on enhancing the skills, knowledge and social capabilities available to individuals, institutions and social and political systems'. Nancy Gerein, in her chapter on capacity development, talks about the evolution of this field over the last 50 years from theory to its current state in meeting the strategic needs of health management and capacity requirements (at the individual, organisational, social and global levels). She argues that the framework for capacity development should focus on both top-down and bottom-up approaches. The process of capacity development for health management involves capacity assessment at every level, identifying gaps and thereby formulating strategies for achieving the required capacities. Training is one of the most important parts of capacity development for government, large organisations, small businesses and civil society organisations.

Keerti Bhusan Pradhan in his chapter 'Capacity Development Model in Enhancing Health Care (EYE CARE) Services—The Aravind Eye Care Model', indicates that it is a unique business model with strong organisational culture base on spirituality. The Aravind Eye Care Model is one of the best examples of capacity development in India. Aravind Hospital has 4,000 beds and performs more than 250,000 eye surgeries per year. It is perhaps the world's largest provider of eye care services. Its range of services varies from very strong community outreach programmes to world class clinical services and dissemination. It offers 65 per cent of its services free without compromising on quality. The Aravind Model has been extended to hospitals in a large number of countries in Latin America, Africa and Asia.

National health programmes

Rajeev Sadanandan discusses the issues involved in 'Managing AIDS Control Programme in India'. Various challenges involved in implementing the AIDS control programme are the stigma of epidemic drivers, mainstreaming with other sectors and health programmes, integration of different AIDS programmes and so on. High order programming, technical support, human resources and use of strategic information for planning and mid-course correction are other issues involved in programme implementation. The new phase proposes to scale up the programme with greater emphasis on treatment and impact mitigation. There will be also greater emphasis on public-private partnerships, decentralisation at district level, dedicated strategic information management units, involvement of national and regional institutions of excellence in capacity building and arrangements to support programme implementation in states that have underperformed in the past.

Dileep Mavalankar in his chapter on National Rural Health Mission (NRHM) outlines its underlying vision, concept, core strategies and activities. NRHM objectives focus on improvements in maternal health, fertility reduction and disease control by 2012. NRHM proposes to change the basic structure of health care delivery system in India. It focuses on overall improvement in health, rather than only reproductive and child health. The key concept in NRHM is to bring all the health and family welfare programmes, including Reproductive and Child Health (RCH-II), under one umbrella. The objectives of NRHM are to be achieved through six core strategies, that is, (*a*) establishing community health workers called ASHA; (*b*) infrastructure improvements; (*c*) capacity building; (*d*) private-public partnership; (*e*) risk pooling and social health insurance; and (*f*) decentralised planning.

Maternal and child health

On the subject of 'Achieving the Millennium Development Goals for Maternal and Newborn Health', Ardi Kaptiningsih says that every country, either with high level or low level of skilled care at birth, is facing challenges in maternal and neonatal mortality reduction. For example, countries with less than 50 per cent skilled care at birth are dealing with competing priorities to improve access and quality of care. Countries with medium level of skilled attendance (between 50 per cent and 80 per cent) need to strengthen logistical and referral system and quality of care. On the contrary, countries with greater than 80 per cent skilled birth attendance need to reduce over-medicalisation in normal pregnancy and childbirth. Therefore, policy issues related to human resource development and management, capacity development, financing, referral system, quality of services, effective coordination with individuals, families and communities, and multi-sectoral and inter-country collaborations become critical.

Urvashi Chandra and Sangeeta Singh bring out the critical need for community participation for effective service delivery in their chapter on the role of community participation for maternal and child health. This chapter discusses two case studies, one each from Chattisgarh and Haryana. There are ample evidences to show that working with village health workers and community groups at the grassroot level leads to community empowerment, particularly of women. *Mitanins* in Chhattisgarh and *Sanjeevanis* in Haryana are two good examples of community participation under the European Commission's Sector Investment Programme. Community ownership plays an important role in the sustainability of effective health care delivery system, and therefore the process of selection of these 'change agents' is critical. Forging strong partnerships between communities and health services so as to meet the increased demand for services with improved supply, is crucial for attaining the goals for better health.

Urban health

In their chapter on public-private partnership in managing urban health, K. V. Ramani et al. outline the approach to develop a PPP model for a decentralised and integrated primary health care centre for Ahmedabad city. This model is based on a Geographic Information Systems (GIS) analysis to identify a good location and ensure availability, access, affordability and equity in the provision of primary health services. The model has been successfully applied to one ward in Ahmedabad city, namely, Vasna ward. It is built on a clear understanding of the socio-economic profile, status of public health, and the health care seeking habits of the Vasna population. A partnership between the Ahmedabad Municipal Corporation (AMC), Gujarat Cancer Society (GCS), Akhand Jyot Foundation (Service provider NGO) and SAATH (Community NGO) has been established. This model is now under consideration by the AMC for replication in all the wards of Ahmedabad city.

Communicable diseases

Michael Friedman, in his chapter on the need to improve the standards of medical care in India, focuses on the quality HIV care in Indian medical institutions. Multiple creative strategies are necessary to provide quality care, improve the knowledge of medical professionals, implement penalties for poor quality medical practices, revoke medical licenses or hospital privileges and terminate form services. Creating an accreditation system based on a set of standards of care can be an effective tool for ensuring excellent service quality. The Revised National TB Control Programme (RNTCP) may be considered a good example to demonstrate the effectiveness of clearly defined standards of care.

There is an attempt to establish HIV care standards similar to the standards of care for other diseases. However, there are several issues for accreditation of HIV care services, such as identification of the best model of HIV care, limited number of accreditation agencies, and the demand for HIV care services because of its sensitivity. Friedman concludes with the lines of Mager, 'If you are not certain of where you are going...you may very well end up somewhere else (and not even know it)'.

Non-communicable diseases

A. Nandakumar in his chapter 'Challenges and Approaches towards the Control of Chronic Diseases in a Developing Country with Cancer as a Model' has taken the example of cancer. Developing a cancer atlas involves continuous and systematic data collection on the occurrence and characteristics of various types of cancer in different parts of the country. In India, the National Cancer Registry programme started in 1981 and as of now there are 21 population-based and five hospital-based cancer registries. An analysis of the cancer data gives new insights into cancer incidence and prevalence patterns with the identification of areas with high incidence, recognised geographical belts of various types of cancer, and discerned likely zones. He demonstrates the immense potential of cancer atlas data reporting system and the numerous possibilities for cancer research and control.

A. Vaidheesh in his chapter discusses the 'Health Care Delivery Challenges for Chronic Diseases in India'. Lifestyle diseases such as obesity, cardiovascular diseases and diabetes are growing enormously. In spite of high incidence of such diseases, interventions have been slow and delayed, mainly due to insufficient medical infrastructure such as screening programmes, trained surgeons, interventional physicians and general practitioners. Low awareness, ignorance, fear and affordability prevent many people from undergoing regular check-ups. There is a shortage of super speciality hospitals in the public sector and therefore it may be advisable to explore partnerships with private hospitals to respond to the challenges in the treatment of non-communicable diseases.

Scaling up Health in Low Income Settings

1

Jeffrey D. Sachs

It is commonly understood that India needs a major push for public health improvement. India is currently making economic advances that should also be translated into advances in the public health system, which is currently inadequate. Instead, public health advances are lagging behind the process of overall economic development, to the extent that the failure to advance health actually threatens economic progress. In 2000–01, the Commission on Macroeconomics and Health (CMH), which I chaired, was established to look at the interactions between health and economic development. Within CMH, a sub-committee on CMH in India was formed to focus on India's unique situation. CMH first identified three major topics for investigation: the role of health in overall economic progress; the general conditions that low income countries face and that present the biggest challenges to public health; and finally, developing solutions for resolution of these challenges. I will address these topics first on a broad, global level, and will then concentrate specifically on the challenges that India faces.

The first conclusion of CMH was that health is in many ways a major spur to overall economic development. Improved health leads to greater individual productivity, greater investment in human capital, better education and better on-the-job training, all of which produce a more highly skilled labour force. Combined, these improvements result in a more rapid and sound demographic transition from a high birth rate to a low birth rate. Reduction of the total fertility rate is itself a major input of economic development. As economists have long noted, when poor families move from having five or six children to having just two children, higher levels of investment can be made per child in terms of nutrition, health care and education. Thus, investing in health is a major asset, not only in well-being, but also in economic development; while poverty leads to bad health, bad health also is a factor in the continuation of poverty.

Next, the Commission tried to ascertain the main conditions that low income countries face with regard to the gap in their health conditions compared to those of high income countries. In this situation, individual circumstances define a country's position. India finds itself somewhere between Sub-Saharan African countries which have poor health indicators and high-income countries which have good health indicators. And, within India, there are vast differences in health conditions—southern states, such as Kerala, have relatively better health conditions than the Gangetic north, where states like Uttar Pradesh and Bihar have some of the worst health conditions, not just in India but also relative to the rest of the world. The Commission found that, on an average, low income countries face a high preponderance of infectious disease challenges, such as HIV/AIDS, tuberculosis, malaria, respiratory infections and diarrheal diseases. Other conditions, like macro- and micronutrient deficiencies, parasitic infections like helminths and maternal and peri-natal deaths remain a major consideration. The infectious disease burden and maternal conditions remain serious problems, especially since India increasingly suffers from a 'dual-disease' burden. Not only does it suffer from the traditional infectious diseases just mentioned, but it is also experiencing an increase in the incidence of chronic diseases such as adult onset diabetes, metabolic disorders resulting from the 'modern lifestyle' shift to high fat intakes (which very surprisingly is affecting India a great deal), cardio-vascular disease, and the largely undiagnosed and untreated hypertension. In general, health statistics of India are not good: life expectancy is between 63 and 64 years, infant mortality rate is around 70 per 1,000 live births, the under-five mortality rate is 100 per 1,000 live births, and the maternal mortality ratio is estimated to be around 400 per 100,000 live births. The latter ratio is one of the highest in the world and clearly indicates that women are not attended to properly in their sexual health needs or in safe childbirth. Undernourishment still afflicts perhaps 40–50 per cent of Indian children and it is reported that up to 40–50 per cent of mothers have anemia. So, conditions are of course better than they used to be in India and better than in many impoverished sub-Saharan African countries, but the present conditions are still not where India ought to be, considering the economy's dramatic, multi-sectoral progress.

So what can we do about it? Solutions are complicated, as good health depends partly on the health system and partly on the general environment, both social and infrastructural, in which people live. First, it is important to understand the environmental factors that affect people's health. We know that health is determined in part by access to safe drinking water, sanitation (a very important component which is woefully lacking in rural India), literacy and education, and by access to basic services such as transportation and electricity. Ethnic and gender equity is also a key factor, as access to health services for women is often restricted both within the broader society and within the household, as seen when husbands or mothers-in-law do not allow their pregnant wives or daughters-in-law to receive proper treatment. Scheduled castes, scheduled tribes and other minority groups face similar discrimination and restrictions. All of these components play a role in shaping health outcomes, and so too does the health system itself.

In making the proper diagnosis of Indian health care, the CMH studied in detail, the kind of health system that is needed to address essential health needs in a low income setting. The Commission found that the Indian health system actually looks more or less right. On paper, India has a whole hierarchy of health services, which are provided by both the state and federal government, starting at the lowest rural level with sub-centres and moving to primary health centres, community health centre, district hospitals, state hospitals and finally to national units at the highest level. This is the kind of system the Commission believed in: a public health system that had an organised hierarchy right from the village to the union level. However, in moving from the on-paper theory to actual practice in India, the CMH found a dreadful gap. In determining the cause for this, CMH asked the question: 'How much does it cost to run a proper health system?' And it was here that the biggest problem with India's health care was found. In 2001, when CMH wrote the report, or even today in 2005, it cost about 35–40 US dollars per person per year, to establish a proper public health system. However, in India, spending on public health through both the state and federal budgets is still only about 1 per cent of the GNP, or about 5 US dollars per person per year in public health spending. This amount is so small that the whole Indian hierarchy, from the sub-centres to Community Health Centres (CHCs), is essentially dysfunctional. Often, staff are not present, nor are record-keeping, medicines, running water, electricity, or phones. Because of the huge gap between 5 US dollars and 35 US dollars, the theoretically excellent system on paper cannot work in practice.

Of course, the result in India is that people at all income levels avoid the state-run system and instead go to private providers. Unfortunately, evidence shows that the quality of private care is terrible—private providers are poorly educated, trained, equipped and monitored. And, it is an expensive system because the poor pay out of pocket for health care, as they have no insurance and as a result must often sell vital assets such as cattle or farm equipment in order to obtain emergency health care. Large sacrifices are made with very meager results. Some experts have concluded that what India really needs is a strong private health system, as 5/6th of all spending is already done in the private health system. The CMH found decisively that such logic is wrong. People go to private providers because the public sector is deficient, but that is not a reason to give up on the public sector. The private sector does not provide adequate help for the health of the overall population, and especially for the poor, nor can it do so. The poor need a publicly provided system that is reliable and will give quality care, because they cannot afford to pay for adequate care out of pocket. To leave the poor to fend for themselves in the private sector will not lead to proper health outcomes, and to conclude that a private system should be India's system because 5/6th of spending occurs there is simply a measure of defeat, not of good reason.

So, CMH made several recommendations for improving the Indian public health system for provision of essential health services. First and foremost, the level of financing must be scaled up, but not arbitrarily. Instead, economic financing must be done in a way that will address the complex governance challenges that are faced by a country as vast as India. So, the first recommendation is implementation of 'close-to-client systems' that are actually similar to Indian sub-centres and Primary Health Centres (PHCs), but would instead have the proper investments: each with electricity, refrigeration systems for medicines, running water, telecommunications and some kind of ambulance service for village populations (about 5,000 people). This is achievable in India, especially with its brilliant use of Information Technology (IT) in achieving the growing connectedness of villages. Also, politics demands services in rural areas, and this was the main message of the last election and is considered to be the National Common Minimum Programme of the Government of India (May 2004). However, even with political support, India does not see proper investment occurring at the rural level.

As a result, policy makers must develop creative reforms, especially focusing on establishing proper Village-Based Workers (VBWs). Perhaps a whole cadre of VBW with a year or two of training should be established to address basic needs: malaria, TB identification and control of diarrheal disease. These VBWs could also provide community aid so that women would get either the appropriate antenatal care or would be rushed to an appropriate facility for emergency delivery if hemorrhage, sepsis, or other potentially fatal conditions occur. Village-based Workers (VBW) and the proper local facilities need local oversight, however, and a system for monitoring must be implemented at the local level. This could potentially be the role of village-based panchayats, as some success has been seen thus far with their leadership in overseeing health and education sectors, but such successes are largely local, occurring in Kerala but not in the poor, populous states of northern India.

It is striking that India has not really taken on this challenge politically or analytically—there are no proper schools of public health to study disease burden in India state by state and sector by sector. Nor is there a school that could analyse the role of the non-health sector input (water, literacy, transport, communications, ethnic and gender equality) as well as the public health system itself (system organisation, cost, financing and political involvement). It is imperative to develop a rigorous, comprehensive and systematic study of the disease burden, epidemiological challenges and the organisation of the public health system in order to achieve important breakthroughs.

All over India there are small-scale success stories of treating key infectious diseases, of panchayats using local delivery of services and of actually diagnosing and treating chronic diseases (that is, high blood pressure, which can be treated at low cost but remains almost undiagnosed in rural and poor urban areas). We need to study, along with broad epidemiological analysis, the success stories taking place in many districts, regions, and NGOs. These successes must be brought to the national scale and the imperative of scaling up health systems as a priority matter must be emphasised to health ministers and the leadership throughout the union. The public demands it, politics demands it and the economy absolutely demands it. This is really the decade when India should face up to and finally conquer the extreme poverty in its midst, and this is now possible with India's dynamism, leadership, IT capabilities and economic and social vigour. This decade should be the breakthrough decade for India on all fronts in the fight against extreme poverty: for reducing the burden of disease, for raising life expectancies, for saving mothers now dying during childbirth and for cutting sharply the child and infant mortality rates. The levels of success that are achieved in states like Tamil Nadu and Kerala should be achieved all over India—this is really the essential task.

Health Systems: A 2020 Vision

2

Andrew Green

Background

This chapter addresses the future challenges to health systems with respect to contextual changes at the global and national levels. Understanding the historical evolution of health systems is necessary to understand the current health situation.

Post Alma Ata

The earlier Alma Ata declaration (WHO 1978) focussed on developing primary health care policies, but by the end of the 1980s, this approach was perceived to have failed to improve health. Health indicators reflected the growing gap between wealthy and poor economies and an assessment of global health in the early 1990s revealed poor health outcomes for many developing countries, including India (see Table 2.1). During the 1990s, the worldwide Under-Five Mortality Rate (U5MR) was 96 deaths per 1,000 children under 5 years old and the global life expectancy at birth was 65 years. However, the U5MR rate documented in Sub-Saharan Africa (SSA) was 175 deaths per 1,000 children, in India it was 127 deaths per 1,000 children, and both India and SSA experienced some of the lowest life expectancies at birth in the world. Health expenditure comprised only a small percentage of the GDP (the global average was 323 US dollars per capita), and the per capita health expenditure was as low as 11 US dollars in China and 21 US dollars in India.

Table 2.1 **Key indicators of resources and health needs, 1990**

Countries/Regions	Health expenditure		Child mortality rate (under-five mortality rate per 1,000 children)	Life expectancy at birth (years)
	Per capita (in US dollars)	As % of GDP		
Sub-Saharan Africa	24	4.5	175	52
India	21	6	127	58
China	11	3.5	43	69
Other Asian Countries and Islands	61	4.5	97	62
Latin America and Caribbean	105	4	60	70
Middle Eastern Crescent	77	4.1	111	61
Formerly Socialist Economies of Europe	142	3.6	22	72
Established Market Economies	1,860	9.6	11	76
World	323	8	96	65

Source: World Bank 1993.

These gaps in health resources and failures in addressing health needs led to 'reforms' in health system structures.

Health sector reforms—why and what?

The movement for public health system reform began in the early 1990s. At that time, as has been seen, the health system was struggling to achieve health gains. This was perceived by many as the result of over-bureaucratisation, centralisation, system-wide inefficiency and insensitivity to change within the public sector. This resulted in disillusionment with the public sector and a growing belief that structural change in the public health system was needed. Linked to this was a wider ideological shift to the 'new right', which argued for a minimal role for government. Policy makers and agencies, and in particular the World Bank, identified three broad areas for reform. The first focussed on the structure and governance of the health system. Specifically, an attempt was made to change the government's role in the health system from that of the traditional provider to one that sets policy, regulates and commissions other groups to provide health care service. As part of this shift, the private sector, both profit and non-profit, began to have a greater role and influence in the provision of health care, resulting in the introduction of private sector management approaches in the public sector. Structural changes also included moves to decentralise decision-making within the public sector and in some areas the integration of vertical programmes into general service delivery.

The second area for reform involved the low level of resources and the resulting necessity of developing and creating new mechanisms for revenue. In the 1990s, emphasis was placed on user fees paid by health care consumers as a means of raising revenue. However, the lack of resources in the government sector, even after implementation of user fees, reinforced the need for priority-setting as the third area for reform. The focus shifted to developing 'minimum care' packages. Economic approaches and techniques for assessing cost-effectiveness emerged along side traditional epidemiological practices.

Underpinning the reforms were various assumptions which were often not explicit. It was assumed that competition amongst providers would enhance efficiency; that there was an inevitability in the public sector's bureaucratic and unresponsive nature that inherently results in inefficiency; that a consumerist rather than community view was appropriate; and finally, that focus should be given to personal responsibility for financing via user charges rather than collective financing. It is important to remember, however, that all these assumptions are just that—assumptions and not evidence-based statements—and can be challenged.

Criticisms of health sector reforms

By the end of the 1990s, the reforms had attracted criticism from academics and policy makers. They were seen to have focussed on supply-side issues without giving due attention to the demands and the needs of community and individual health. They were also criticised for emphasising the health *sector* rather than health *care*. Furthermore, insufficient attention was given to regulating the private sector or creating public-private partnerships to link the health sector with other sectors and agencies. An overly technocratic and narrow prioritisation strategy was criticised for its concentration on diseases rather than wider health. The focus of the reforms on structures was also seen as ignoring critical human resource issues. Finally, despite user charges, low levels of health financing and funding led to major difficulties for the health system, not least because of policy concerns about the inequity of user charges and their discriminatory effect on vulnerable and poor populations.

Concerns were also voiced over the actual process of developing these reforms. Many reforms were adopted without proper evidence to support their implementation. Reforms were also largely instigated by external partners, often with financial leverage, resulting in a lack of local ownership. 'Blueprintism' was a major failure, as it ignored the importance of contextual sensitivity. This is especially evident in a country like India, where context differs not only in respect to other countries, but also internally, with variance from state to state. The reforms also appeared to coincide with an apparent decline in the public sector ethos and values with the possibility that this was a consequence of the reforms.

Though it is perhaps artificially convenient to see significant shifts with the new millennium, a number of such shifts can, coincidentally perhaps, be identified. By the end of the 1990s, a shift away from a single set of reforms can be discerned. Despite its controversial attempt to develop a single measure and league table for health systems (see Table 2.2), the WHO 2000 Report on Health Systems set out a model for understanding health systems which encouraged a focus on performance rather than structure alone. The setting up of the WHO Commission on Social Determinants of Health also indicated growing recognition of the importance of policies on wider determinants of health, building on earlier WHO work on tobacco. The need for better evidence-based policy-making was a key theme in the WHO conference on health systems in Mexico.

Table 2.2   Health system attainment and performance, ranked by eight measures, estimates for 1997—selected countries

Member state	Health attainment		Responsiveness of health system		Fairness in financial contribution	Overall health system goal attainment	Health expenditure per capita in international $	Health system performance	
	Level (DALE)	Distribution (Equality of child survival)	Level	Distribution				On health level	Overall performance
France	3	12	16-17	3-38	26-29	6	4	4	1
Italy	6	14	22-23	3-38	45-47	11	11	3	2
Oman	72	59	83	49	56-57	59	62	1	8
Japan	1	3	6	3-38	8-11	1	13	9	10
UK	14	2	26-27	3-38	08-11	9	26	24	18
Germany	22	20	5	3-38	6-7	14	3	41	25
USA	24	32	1	3-38	54-55	15	1	72	37
Senegal	151	105	118-9	104	87	118	143	132	59
Bangladesh	140	125	178	181	51-52	131	144	103	88
Indonesia	103	156	63-64	70	73	106	154	90	92
Iran	96	113	100	93-94	112-113	114	94	58	93
India	134	153	108-10	127	42-44	121	133	118	112

(Table 2.2 continued)

(Table 2.2 continued)

| Member state | Health attainment | | Attainment of goals | | | | | Health expenditure per capita in international $ | Health system performance | |
| | Level (DALE) | Distribution (Equality of child survival) | Responsiveness of health system | | Fairness in financial contribution | Overall health system goal attainment | | | On health level | Overall performance |
			Level	Distribution						
Pakistan	124	183	120–1	115	62–63	133	142		85	122
Ghana	149	149	132–5	146	74–75	139	166		158	135
China	81	101	88–9	105–6	188	132	139		61	144
165	186	138	187–8		128–130	162	168		179	149
Nepal	142	161	185	166–7	186	160	170		98	150
Tanzania	176	172	157–60	150	48	158	174		180	156
Afghanistan	168	182	181–2	172–3	103–104	183	184		150	173
South Africa	160	128	73–74	147	142–143	151	57		182	175
Sierra Leone	191	186	173	186	191	191	183		183	191

Source: WHO 2000.

There was also increasing recognition of the critical constraints placed on countries by the low levels of resources, either due to general low economic development or, as in the case of countries such as India, due to the low priority given by the public sector to health. Table 2.3 depicts the level and sources of health funding in selected countries and clearly shows the differences in health care spending and sources. In a situation of chronically low levels of resources, restructuring of services is unlikely to be productive and may indeed be diversionary. The Committee on Macro-Economics and Health (CMEH), established in 2000, analysed the low levels of current health financing and the subsequent need for exploring alternate funding sources. Unlike higher income nations, where the majority of health expenditure comes from tax or social security, developing nations such as Ethiopia, Uganda and India, finance health expenditures primarily out of pocket. Among these nations, India has the highest percentage of out-of-pocket spending. During 2000, total per capita expenditure at the official exchange rate was just 23 US dollars in India as

Table 2.3   Levels and sources of finance—selected countries

Countries	Total per capita health expenditure at official exchange rate (US$)	Total expenditure on health as percentage of GDP	Per cent of total expenditure by source			
			Tax	Social security	Private other than out of pocket	Out of pocket
Ethiopia	4	3.8	36.2	0.0	0.0	63.8
Uganda	14	4.1	35.0	0.0	16.7	48.2
India	23	5.2	13.0	n.a.	2.4	84.6
Cuba	131	6.3	87.5	0.0	0.0	12.5
Thailand	133	5.7	29.3	3.7	1.6	65.4
Argentina	676	8.2	22.8	34.7	9.9	32.6
UK	1,303	5.8	96.9	0.0	0.0	3.1
France	2,369	9.8	2.5	74.4	2.7	20.4
USA	4,187	13.7	25.5	18.6	39.3	16.6

Source: WHO 2000.

compared to 4,187 US dollars in the US. There is also increasing recognition of the deficiencies of aid architecture and in some cases, shifts towards sectoral rather than project support through mechanisms such as Sector Wide Approaches (SWAs).

With the new millennium also came a growing recognition of an impending human resource crisis globally and already occurring in some low income countries. It is, for example, estimated that an additional 334,000 midwives will be required in the next 10 years (WHO 2005). Exacerbating the difficulties in particular countries is a growth in international migration of skilled workers from developing to developed nations, attributable to a variety of complex push and pull reasons, including the low morale of staff in developing nations. This, of course, is leading to even wider inequities in distribution of human resources between richer and poorer countries, as shown in Figure 2.1.

Figure 2.1   Supply of nurses and midwives per 100,000 population—selected countries

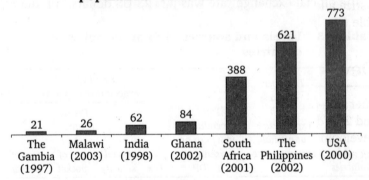

Another trend can be discerned in the last decade—the growing role of NGOs in advocacy issues over international issues. The International Conference on Population and Development in Cairo in 1994 was an early example of the growing importance of NGOs in influencing international policy. A more recent example is the publication of the Global Health Watch (People's Health Movement 2005) as an alternative perspective to the WHO annual World Health Report.

The millennium was marked by the UN with a set of Development Goals for 2015 pledged by its members. The goals created targets for eradicating extreme poverty and hunger, achieving universal primary education, promoting gender equality and empowering women, reducing child mortality, improving maternal health, combating infectious diseases such as HIV/AIDS and malaria, ensuring environmental sustainability and establishing global development partnerships. However, progress to date, particularly in Sub-Saharan Africa, has been disappointing. According to the UN, if current trends continue, the worldwide reduction in under-five mortality would be just 15 per cent between 1990 and 2015, which is well short of the target of two-thirds reduction. Estimates continue to indicate high maternal mortality ratios in Sub-Saharan Africa and southern Asia. Though significant declines have occurred in countries with moderate to low levels of maternal mortality, similar progress cannot be discerned in high-mortality settings. Because of the inadequacy of the health system, particularly in rural areas, many women are still dying during childbirth. The reduction in the number of maternal deaths is not only a health issue but is an issue of social justice and human rights, as most of these deaths are preventable (see http://unstats.un.org/unsd/mi/mi_coverfinal.htm).

Developing a health system for 2020

After a brief discussion of few key indicators (mentioned in Tables 2.2 and 2.3) during last two decades, there is a need to look at the development of a 'fit for purpose' health system for the next two decades. It basically focuses on the three issues,

1. What will be the context?
2. What will be the needs of health?
3. What needs should be addressed related to health system needs?

Emerging contextual issues

We first look at a number of contextual issues and likely changes that may occur over the next two decades, starting with globalisation.

Globalisation

There are a number of ways in which globalisation is likely to affect national health systems.

First, it is a trite but true statement that ill-health does not need a visa and we are increasingly seeing the transmission of diseases among countries, and indeed regions, in a way that suggests a stronger need for international co-operation in disease control.

Second, there is a growth in international migration of skilled personnel, which has already been referred to. It seems likely that this will, if anything, increase rather than decline in future years, again leading to the need for both international action and regulation, and for individual national health systems to recognise and respond to international trends in this area.

Third, it is currently unclear what the impact of the negotiations led by the World Trade Organization (WTO) are likely to be within the health sector, but it would appear that the commodification of health and increased marketisation is likely to see the development of multinational health providers and an increase in the shift of patients between countries. Commercial international interests are also likely to continue to be an important contextual element for health systems in the way that we have already experienced with pharmaceutical multinationals.

Conflict among nations clearly has an impact on health and although it is hard to measure whether this is increasing or is being better reported, it would be naive to assume that international conflict will disappear.

Finally, it appears likely that globalisation will also affect the expectations of users about their own rights and about the rights of communities as a whole, and this, linked with stronger advocacy mechanisms and wider information technology, suggests that professional services such as health are likely to have to learn new ways of responding to a greater rights-based agenda.

Governance

We see an increasing interest in the role of governance within the heath sector, with issues such as how decisions are made, how accountable professionals are to the wider society, the role of civil society in making decisions, and the negative effects of corruption becoming areas of policy concern. One particular aspect that was pushed in the 1990s was decentralisation, and this is likely to continue. However, at the other extreme, it is also possible that, given the global trends that we have seen, inter-country regional bodies may be set up to co-ordinate national responses.

Global economic and political shifts

We are clearly seeing significant geopolitical and economic shifts occurring in the world, with most obviously the decline in the influence of the former USSR and rise in the power of India and China. The implications of this are likely to be huge, both in terms of economic shifts and in terms of how, this, then relates to health patterns and to governance of international bodies.

Crises—natural and artificial

We have already referred in the previous section to war; other forms of crises are also likely to continue, including natural disasters (such as the Tsunami or famines), or artificial disasters like political instability within a country (such as currently in Zimbabwe).

Urbanisation

Thirty years ago the main emphasis in health systems was on provision of care for disadvantaged rural communities in low income countries. Whilst this clearly remains an important objective, increasing urbanisation occurring globally suggests the need for us to consider, alongside rural deprivation, the real needs of urban populations and the best way in which health systems can be designed to cater to their needs.

Environmental degradation

As we continue to experience degradation of the environment, and in particular the warming of the planet, this is likely to have knock-on effects within the health field, ranging from the potential for more natural disasters through shifts in economies to indeed, different patterns of ill-health.

Technology and health care

Technology is advancing and shifting on what appears, an almost daily basis, and this is bound to have an impact on health systems over the next two decades. Three particular examples of technology change can be identified, including the whole development of the technology of genetic medicine, the use of telemedicine techniques and the use of information technology for decision-making.

Consumer expectations

I have already referred to probable changes in consumer expectations and there are three areas that are likely to affect this. First, growth in information technology will influence consumer consciousness and information sharing. This, coupled with greater interest in rights-based approaches to medicine, is likely to lead to greater consumerism and community action around medical issues. One danger with this is that the health system will respond defensively to this, as we see, for example, the type of defensive medicine practices, in particular, the American health system.

Health needs in the future

The second broad area relates to the likely health needs in 2020 and Table 2.4 sets out projections concerning the rank order of disease burden for 15 leading causes, showing the shifts that are regarded as likely to occur. Without looking at the details of this, it is clear that certain health problems are likely to become more important, implying the need for changes in the type of health system and services provided. The trends within this which are well recognised as occurring include the impact of changing demography in populations, together with a growth in non-communicable diseases; potentially new emerging communicable diseases such as HIV/AIDS and Avian Flu; and greater importance to what we currently class as 'neglected diseases'.

Table 2.4   Rank order of disease burden for 15 leading causes

Disease or injury 1990	Rank	Disease or injury 2020
Lower respiratory infections (pneumonia)	1	Ischaemic heart disease
Diarrhoeal diseases	2	Unipolar major depression
Perinatal (newborn) conditions	3	Road traffic accidents
Unipolar major depression	4	Cerebrovascular disease (stroke)
Ischaemic heart disease	5	Chronic obstructive pulmonary disease
Cerebrovascular disease	6	Lower respiratory infections
Tuberculosis	7	Tuberculosis
Measles	8	War
Road traffic accidents	9	Diarrhoeal diseases
Congenital anomalies	10	HIV
Chronic obstructive pulmonary disease	11	Perinatal conditions
Malaria	12	Violence
Falls	13	Congenital anomalies
Iron deficiency anaemia	14	Self-inflicted injuries
Protein-energy malnutrition	15	Trachea, bronchus and lung cancer

Source: Adapted from http://healthlink.mcw.edu/article/977858884.html Accessed.

Health system responses

All the above is likely to need particular health system responses and in an article of this length it is impossible to go into these in any detail. However, to illustrate the type of responses, a number of broad areas are outlined further.

General expansion of services

It is likely that services will need to expand due to the pressure of expectations and the changing needs. However, it is also important that the health system recognises that some services may be able to be downsized as health needs change.

Types of health care offered

The health system will need to make decisions regarding the sorts of health care provided. These are exemplified here.

1. The balance between urban, rural and peri-urban services
2. The balance between chronic and acute care
3. The balance between care provided in institutions versus care provided at home
4. Mechanisms for improving referral between systems
5. The importance of developing integrated care and care pathways
6. The balance between services that attempt to cure and services that provide care
7. The service implications of growing tele-medicine
8. International responses to crises and cross-border health issues.

A number of these will also lead to critical ethical issues in areas such as euthanasia, reproductive health, cloning and use of organs.

Ownership and roles of health agencies

How health care is offered is also likely to be of increasing interest, with potentially a greater role for the private and NGO sectors in systems that have been largely public sector dominated. There is also likely to be greater international trading in health care through multinational corporations, all suggesting the need for greater co-ordination and regulation of health services.

Types of health professionals

The changes are also likely to lead to shifts in the types of health professionals, with greater emphasis on particular competencies needed rather than professional groupings and hence less demarcation between professional roles with the services being generic at the point of the patient. International migration is also likely to lead to attempts by countries to develop auxiliary cadres which do not have international marketability. This will have implications for the types of training models that are currently used.

Economic implications

The inequities of resources between countries and the greater internationalisation described above also suggest that there is likely to be more push, both on a pragmatic and on a moral ground, for greater transfer of resources from rich nations to poorer nations rather than the reverse. However, mechanisms for this are clearly politically fraught.

Community engagement models

How communities engage with the health service is also likely to change with different governance models, and this is likely to be both at the individual level in terms of patient/professional inter-relationships and of involvement in clinical care decisions and also at the wider level in terms of areas such as prioritisation approaches.

Management issues

Finally, the health system will have to respond to issues relating to management. This includes potentially new health systems structures (though the lessons of the 1990s need to be remembered) and greater emphasis on quality and performance of management. Information management is likely to become more important, and harnessing the power of information technology will become a greater potential part of management decision-making.

Prioritisation processes are also likely to be increasingly important both in terms of selection of health problems for focus, but also in terms of decisions on adoption of new and often expensive technologies. The health service will need to develop approaches to engage with its users—and perhaps more importantly its non-users. It will also need to develop mechanisms for advocacy towards other sectors in response to recognition of the wider determinants of health.

Finally, health systems are likely to have to more explicitly confront issues of values and prioritisation and of whether priority should be given to extending the length of life or enhancing the quality of life—the conundrum often described as whether to add years to life or life to years.

Multi-sectoral responses

There is also a continued need for greater awareness of multi-sectoral interventions to respond to increasing problems such as road traffic accidents, violence and mental illness.

Conclusion—the emerging challenges

The discussion suggests challenges both at international and national levels for policy makers as we move towards the year 2020. In this final part of the chapter, I would like to pick out some of these for particular consideration.

First, at the international level, I would suggest two particular examples of the need to strengthen the global policy mechanisms. We first need to be creative in developing mechanisms for the regulation of emerging multinational health care providers. We will also need to pay particular attention to the effects of the international competitive framework of the WTO.

Second, international migration can no longer be left to its own devices, but needs some form of international policies and regulations. Third, the aid architecture processes, in particular through the growth of public-private partnerships at the international level, will need concerted international political consideration in terms of the aid framework and the particular mechanisms by which resources are transferred.

There are also, however, a number of challenges for national policy makers. The discussion so far suggests that the health systems of tomorrow will be very different from those that we know today. National policy makers need to look to the future and recognise their responsibility to take control of the design of the health system in a way that we did not see in the 1990s. We need to make health systems work, not just for the provision of health care, but re-orient them to a health promoting agenda, and make them fit for particular national contexts. Particular challenges will be around national human resource policies, given the international migration pressures that are likely to be faced.

National Health Systems also need to look much more closely at how to recapture pride and morale in the public sector, which I would argue will continue to be the driving force for most health systems in low income countries. This suggests also the need to revitalise the capacity of governments to lead the necessary changes and to provide the appropriate regulation and cohesion for fragmented health sectors. The clear resource constraints that face the public sector in health suggests the need for dramatically increased funding, particularly in countries such as India where public health funding is extremely low.

Underpinning all of this is the need for more evidence on health systems, alongside what is often good evidence on the biomedical issues. There is also a need to find mechanisms to manage what is becoming an explosive information management problem.

Finally, I would suggest that health systems need to remind themselves of what I would argue is a critical overall objective— the pursuit of equity of health alongside pragmatism about the means for development.

References

Medical College of Wisconsin. 2003–07. 'Global Health in the 21st Century'. Available online at http://healthlink.mcw.edu/article/ 977858884.html (accessed on December 2005).

People's Health Movement. 2005. *Global Health Watch 2005–06: An Alternative World Health Report*. London: Zed Books.

United Nations Department of Economic Affairs Statistics Division. 'Progress towards the Millennium Development Goals,1990–2005'. Available online at http://mdgs.un.org/unsd/mdg/Resources/ Attach/Products/Progress2005/goal_4.docp.5 (accessed on 7 September 2007).

World Bank. 1993. *World Development Report 1993: Investing in Health.* New York: Oxford University Press.

World Health Organization. 2000. *The World Health Report 2000 Health Systems: Improving Performance.* Geneva: WHO.

———. 2005. *The World Health Report 2005: Make Every Mother and Child Count.* Geneva: WHO.

World Health Organization and the United Nations Children's Fund. 1978. *Report of the International Conference on Primary Health Care. Alma-Ata, USSR, 6–12 September.* Geneva: World Health Organization, (Health for All Series, No. 1).

Equitable Health Financing: A Dream or a Reality?

3

G.N.V. RAMANA

Inequity

The public-subsidy model for health care in India envisaged equitable health care for all Indians. However, the fact remains that such equitable health care still remains a distant goal when inadequate emphasis is placed on systemic accountability. Inequity is clearly visible when the richest segments of society receive the most subsidised health care meant for the poorest. In examining the reason for this disparity, it is evident that the populations with the lowest income levels in society have also the lowest levels of education and awareness. Equity is therefore, a broader universal concept and the health sector can no longer remain disconnected as it has in the past without linkages to any other developmental programmes.

As Figure 3.1 suggests, the lowest income groups receive the smallest share of public subsidies for curative care in India. With increasing income, this share increases. This analysis highlights the failure of the health systems in targeting segments of the society that require public subsidy the most.

The rationale behind providing public subsidy is that there is a group of population that will not have access to basic health, education and nutrition services without active interference by the government. It was thus important for the public health systems to focus on reaching vulnerable groups that need public subsidies the most. However, the findings clearly suggest that strategies to date have failed to do so, and public financing does not reach the poorest populations in reality.

**Figure 3.1   Public financing for curative care in India:
Share of different income groups**

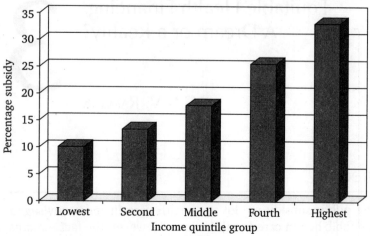

Source: Ajay Mahal et al. 2001.

Global evidence suggests that such inequities in the delivery of
essential health services is widespread among developing countries. A comparative analysis of 56 developing countries undertaken by the World Bank presented in Figure 3.2 shows that the
coverage of basic maternal health services was higher among the
best-off quintile of society as compared to the poorest quintile.
The universality of this inverse trend regarding economic status
and access to health care is observed in oral rehydration therapy,
immunisation, use of modern contraceptives by women and
medical treatment of acute respiratory infections, fever and
diarrhoea. In all cases, a higher percentage of the population is
covered from the richest 20 per cent of the population than the
poorest 20 per cent.

Further substantiating this argument is Figure 3.3, which
depicts how much public subsidy in health care is received by the
richest 20 per cent compared to the poorest 20 per cent. A wide
inter-state variation is evident from this analysis. For example,
in Bihar, a rupee of public subsidy on health care of the poorest
results in subsidy equivalent of rupees 10 taken by the richest.

Figure 3.2 Coverage of basic maternal & health services

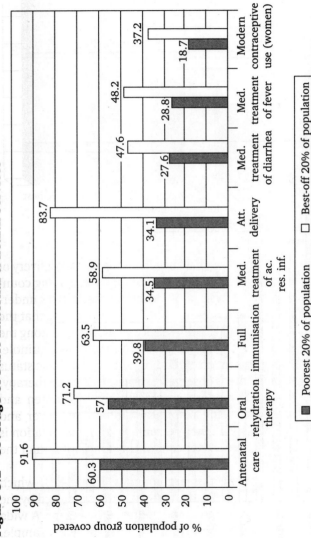

Source: Gwatkin D., Rutstein S., Johnson K, Pande R., Wagstaff A., Socio-economic differences in health, nutrition and population.

Note: Number of countries varies from 51 to 56, depending upon service.

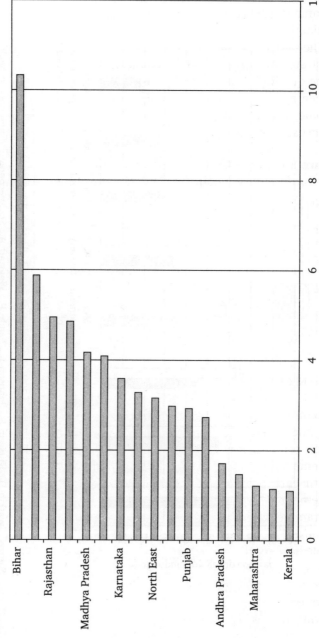

Figure 3.3 Distribution of Indian states by fairness in health financing

That will result in inequitable public health financing. However, in some states like Kerala and Maharashtra such differences are minimal.

The same situation can be seen in another example. Figure 3.4 illustrates coverage of immunisation services as stratified by income quintiles. The analysis shows a direct relationship of the percentage of immunisation achieved with increasing levels of income. The immunisation coverage is marginally better among the urban populations.

Figure 3.4   Inequities in basic immunisation coverage among children (12–23 months) in India

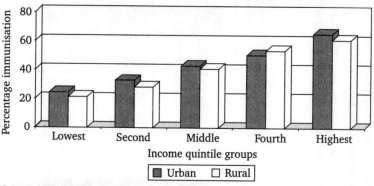

Source: NFHS 1998–99.

Inequity is not confined to a particular country or health system, but instead is a global problem. There are always groups which tend to get overlooked in programme design and implementation and thus remain devoid of benefits from those health care programmes. Even programmes designed and implemented explicitly for the poor are inadequate, as such programmes often fail to target the poorest that need the services the most. Throughout the world, in only four countries the poor people have more access to health services than wealthier populations, and in only two countries the rich and poor have equal access to care. In the rest of the world, wealthy populations obtain more health services. Figure 3.5 depicts the global inequity, showing that the percentage of total expenditure benefiting

Figure 3.5 Inequities in public expenditure on health among 21 developing and transition countries

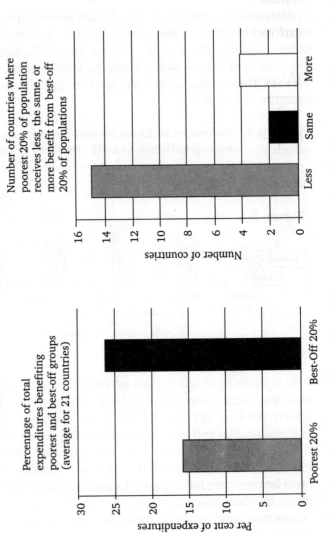

Percentage of expenditures serving the poorest and best-off 20% of the population in 21 developing and transition countries

the poorest population is very little when compared to the percentage benefiting the best-off group. This analysis included 21 transitional and developing nations throughout the world, and serves as an excellent example of worldwide inequities in health care expenditure.

Ways to reach the poor

To reduce or ultimately eliminate inequity and make services pro-poor, programmes and facilities must be targeted better and made more accessible to the poor. There is a broad range of contributions and efforts necessary to achieve this, as shown in Figure 3.6.

Figure 3.6   Inputs for a programme reaching to the poor

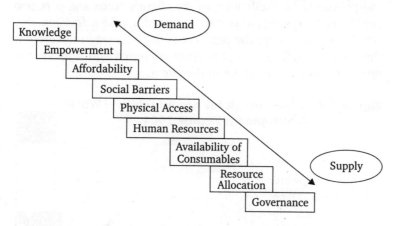

A judicious combination of supply- and demand-side strategies will be required for this. The supply centric approach practised for a long time without fostering any parallel demand from the community has failed to reach the poor. This is because they had no information about the availability of services, or were unaware of the importance of services and above all, were hesitant to use services because of existing social barriers. Thus, without making the atmosphere conducive to use, further increasing the supply will be wasteful. A demand-driven approach will be more appropriate. Complementing the strategies for enhancing demand, is, however, a need to improve the availability of essential services, create accountability mechanisms, empower clients and promote other innovative approaches in service delivery. Some successful models documented from literature covering these aspects are presented here.

Strengthening accountability mechanism

Traditionally, three players are important in service delivery. This includes the client, policy makers and service providers. To date, the accountability mechanisms generally follow a lengthy trajectory that moves from client to policy makers through an electoral process. From the policy makers, the system assigns providers who in turn offer services to the client. This approach has proved to be inefficient, as the client's voice and concerns are lost in the undue amount of time used to take a decision. Direct client power over the provider is the best way to overcome this flawed, ineffective and lengthy approach and it makes the provider more accountable to the client.

Figure 3.7 A framework for accountability: World Development Report 2004

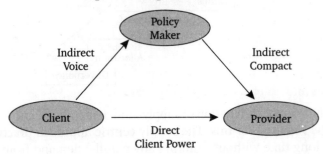

Some of the best examples of strengthening collective accountability are found in an immunisation programme in Tamil Nadu and in decentralisation throughout Madhya Pradesh and Kerala. In Tamil Nadu, the 'fixed day' approach has been successfully adopted, where a policy dictates fixed days on which immunisation services are always made available at health centres. Now many states follow this approach. Through such a policy, accountability gets built into the programme, such that the service is always made available on fixed dates and peer-pressure is used to ensure that the Auxiliary Nurse Midwife (ANM) provides services accordingly. Similarly, all hospitals in Kerala, with the exception of five teaching hospitals, have been handed over to local bodies for administration. Presence of the local panchayat representatives in the hospital advisory committees had a salutary impact on enhancing the accountability of providers to local communities, evidenced by availability of staff and use of services.

Strengthening client power

Typically, clients themselves know the strong and weak points of service delivery the best. Thus, improvement in quality is more likely if clients are empowered with the knowledge and are able to directly monitor and evaluate services. Such client feedback will help in redesigning a programme to be need-based. Various examples of using client contributions to run programmes exist globally and in India as well. In Bangalore, the Citizens Report Card for municipal services, including health and education, was initiated to use client feedback to improve services. A similar client participation programme has also been very successful in the chief minister's mid-day meal programme in Tamil Nadu where parents contribute vegetables and are present for meal preparation. In Mali, there are co-operative pharmacies and user associations that can hire and fire staff. Thus, there are many different ways to strengthen a client's power through empowerment and co-production of services.

Strengthening incentives to providers to serve the poor

Health staff working in rural or remote areas suffer several hardships. Consequently, many of them, especially doctors, are generally reluctant to work in rural areas, as they do not see future progress for their careers, and this reluctance hampers the goal of reaching essential health services to poor rural populations. While providing incentives to the health staff working in rural areas could be a powerful tool for improving services, unfortunately, experiences suggest that doctors are not motivated for such work despite these types of benefits. Other motivational factors are therefore required to make the health staff work for the poor and in rural areas. There are several successful models demonstrated by NGOs such as Karuna Trust in Karnataka which show that it is possible to motivate health providers to reside in rural areas. One successful approach is to train local residents as providers.

Strengthening public-private participation

Traditionally, the government is an important provider of health services, but better programme results can be achieved if the government moves from the role of the provider to that of an active buyer of health outcomes. Governments can be active purchasers through the use of performance-based contracts that work either directly with health providers or through intermediaries. Such an approach is result-oriented and can be better monitored, especially in terms of reaching the poor. However, such policy changes should be made with great caution. Several factors must be seriously considered, including determining which services are to be contracted out, the benefits of contracting, the role and responsibilities of both the buyer and the provider, and appropriate methods to be used for measuring the results and paying incentives.

Such an effort has been made by the government in Andhra Pradesh: basic primary health care, family planning and Reproductive and Child Health (RCH) services in 192 urban health centres and 94 municipalities were contracted out in 2000. This initiative, started under the World Bank-sponsored Urban Slums Project in 2000, is being sustained by the state even after the project closure in 2003. In this project, the government has entered into service contracts with NGOs, including Indian Medical Association (IMA). The NGOs provided the services of a doctor, two ANMs, a helper and a coordinator for an agreed annual compensation while the government provided infrastructure such as buildings, equipment and furniture and ensured constant supply of drugs and other consumables. The self-help groups mobilised communities. The government monitored the project by hiring the services of an independent agency and the results of this programme have kindled hope, as illustrated in Figure 3.8. This programme has achieved a remarkable improvement in the number of pregnant women visited by health workers and also resulted in a salient rise in the number of children fully immunised. However, changes in infant and maternal mortality rates cannot be seen with such short-term programmes, nor is it possible to collect such data from such a small area. Thus, one must be specific and realistic about the changes that can be achieved with short-term programmes. Above all, the advantages of experimenting in urban areas with innovative health care services is that in doing so, the services are made better available to the urban poor.

Sharing information

Information sharing is a powerful tool that increases a client's power and provides a 'short cut' for building accountability. Recently, many hospitals have started creating client charters, which provide information such as bed availability and current stock of essential drugs. This type of information can be used to generate informed debate among clients, who can then decide further action on their own behalf accordingly.

Strengthening demand-side financing

Demand-side financing, where the money following clients, is an emerging novel approach in the social sector. This concept has been tested successfully both in India and abroad. Also known as conditional cash transfers, this is a powerful tool whose success can be best illustrated by two examples. The first is an educational scholarship programme for girls in Bangladesh and the second is PROGRESSA or OPORTUNIDADES, as it is called now, which is an incentive-based poverty alleviation programme for the poor in Mexico. The latter benefits five million families or almost one out of every four Mexicans. This programme actually helps to redistribute public financing towards the poor for short periods of time. Until 1996, various vertical programmes were run for nutrition, health and education and each programme

Figure 3.8 Performances of contracted-out urban health facilities

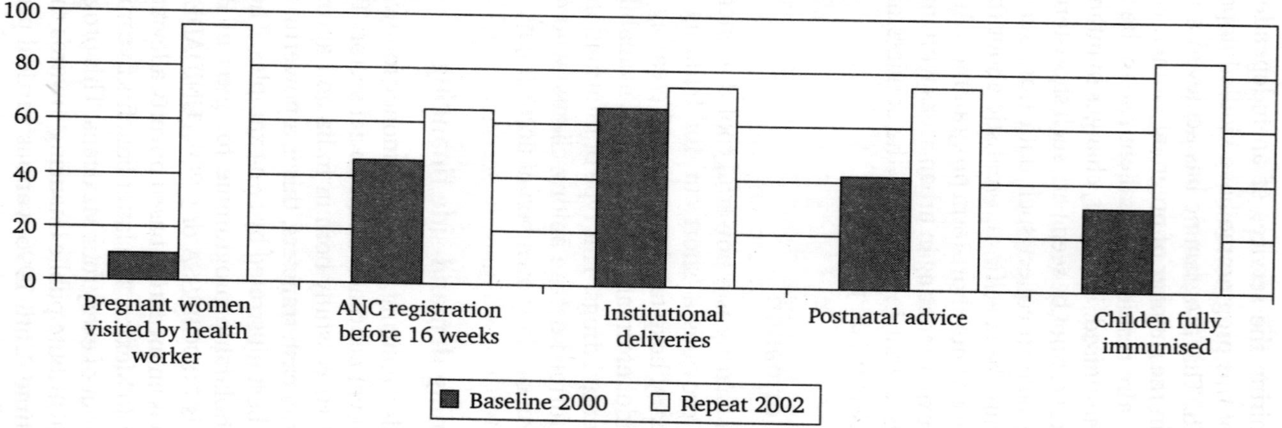

100
80
60
40
20
0

Pregnant women visited by health worker

ANC registration before 16 weeks

Institutional deliveries

Postnatal advice

Childen fully immunised

■ Baseline 2000   □ Repeat 2002

was operated by a separate department, with little to no coordination and zero transparency. Such programmes were not as successful as PROGRESSA due to several problems, like flawed conceptual designs, duplication of efforts, undue bureaucracy, urban/rural imbalances, increasing fiscal resources, general ineffectiveness, burden on government for subsidies and lack of evaluation. PROGRESSA could successfully overcome many of these lacunae using three guiding principles: cash transfers conditional to positive behaviour, co-responsibility in production of services and convergence of the three main dimensions of human development, that is, health, education and nutrition. Three domains are being used in the programme for conditional cash transfers:

1. Nutrition: Nutrition counselling clinics were established for nutritional supplements where mothers could have their children monitored and then receive direct cash incentives.
2. Preventive health care: Cash incentives were given to every member of each family that was enrolled for preventative health care action.
3. School attendance: Children who regularly received/ attended education between third standard in primary school to third standard in secondary school could conditionally be applicants for cash incentives.

The important part of the conditional cash transfer scheme is that cash is deposited to the bank account of the woman in the family. When a woman comes to the clinic, she is explicitly informed that the programme benefits are not conditional to participation in any political event. Another feature of this programme is that even if a family member gets an opportunity for employment, the incentives still continue for three years. Transparency is the biggest strength of this programme: the rules of operation are available on the website, such that one can know exactly how much a specific family receives. Additionally, a list of the number of beneficiary families is published from time to time by the locality, the municipality and the state.

On one hand, the government and families equally share responsibility, while on the other hand, the government has successfully united all three dimensions of human welfare (health, nutrition and education) for the betterment of poor populations and effectiveness of the programme. Figure 3.9 depicts the merger of the three aspects of human welfare.

Target mechanism of OPORTUNIDADES

This programme reaches the neediest populations through effective and transparent targeting mechanisms. It has adopted three steps in this process:

1. Geographical distribution: Geographically targeting rural and poor areas.
2. Eligibility: In the targeted area, eligible households are selected according to pre-determined criteria using census data.
3. Validation: Within each community, the list of selected families is made public and comments are welcomed and received. If a family believes they were unfairly deprived of the facilities, they can submit a second claim to the authorities, the validity of which is then investigated.

Most beneficiaries are agricultural labourers who earn a wage equivalent to 3 US dollars per day.

Monitoring and evaluation

Monitoring and evaluation occurred from the very beginning of the programme as the programme handles the cash transfer process every month and there is intense bimonthly monitoring of indicators. Also, a quasi-experimental design was developed to monitor the impact of the programme. Owing to its intense monitoring and evaluation, the programme has witnessed remarkable impacts, such as a 12 per cent lower incidence of illness among children; reduced probability of stunting among children aged 12–36 months that is equivalent to a 16 per cent increase in average growth rate per year; decrease in iron deficiency anaemia by 18 per cent; 11–14 per cent points increase in secondary school

Figure 3.9 Integrated approach—three closely related and complementary components of human welfare

Family

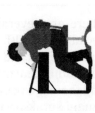

- **Health**
  - preventive actions
  - free basic health package
  - education for hygiene and nutrition
  - measures to strengthen the quality of services

- **Nutrition**
  - cash transfers
  - nutritional supplements for children under five and pregnant and breastfeeding women

  (tied to regular attendance to health centers)

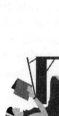

- **Education**
  - scholarships
  - school supplies

  (tied to regular school attendance)

enrolment for girls and 5–8 per cent points for boys; and increase in transition to secondary school by nearly 20 per cent.

Conclusion

There are several approaches to improve access to essential social and health services for the poor. Empowerment of local communities and money could be used as strong incentives for generating demand by providing incentives for positive behaviour, and there are possibilities for replicating similar models in India. Janani Suraksha Yojana (JSY) is a step in this direction—in JSY, women receive monetary incentives for institutional deliveries. However, the main obstacles to such endeavours are leakage and weak or absent monitoring processes. Once these obstacles are removed through improved transparency and robust monitoring systems, India will be able to realistically build such programmes. Additionally, it is crucial to think of innovative methods for public financing. The current government is committed to increasing the public expenditure, and they must be expected to do so—the public expenditure should move from the current 0.9 per cent of the GDP to 1–2 per cent. But still, private out of pocket expenditure on health is going to be high in India and will also increase. With a reality such as this, much flexibility and innovation will be needed for change, but above all, accountability and monitoring must be emphasised if equity is to be achieved in the Indian health care system.

References

Dean Filmer. 2003b. 'The Incidence of Public Expenditure in Health and Education'. Background Paper for the World Development Report 2004.

India-National Family Health Survey. 1998–99. International Institute of Population Sciences, MEASURE DHS+, ORC Macro.

Levine, Ruth and Molly Kinder. 2004. *Millions Saved. Proven Successes in Global Health.* Washington: Centre for Global Development.

Mahal, Ajay, J. Singh, F. Afridi, V. Lamba, A. Gumber and V. Selvaraju. 2002. *Who 'Benefits' from Public Sector Health Spending in India?* New Delhi: National Council for Applied Economic Research.

The World Development Report. 2004. *Making Services Work for the Poor*. World Bank: Oxford University Press.

World Bank Institute. 2005. Reaching the Poor with Health Services, Development Outreach.

World Development Report. 2004. *Making Services Work for Poor People*, The World Bank. Available online at http://econ.worldbank. org/wdr/wder2004/library/doc?id=29478 (accessed on 19 September 2007).

Public-Private Partnership in Health Care

4

MEENAKSHI DATTA GHOSH

Why do we need partnerships?

...Because existing services fail poor people.
...Because the government, on its own, cannot always fully
address the requirements of essential health care for the most
needy populations.

This chapter is an attempt to look at opportunities for possible
Public-Private Partnerships (PPP) in health care as well as their
potential advantages and disadvantages.

Role of the private sector in health care

The idea of PPP has increased in popularity over the past few
years in India. An examination of this term is necessary to understand the actual partnership being proposed. The private sector
has had a growing share in various sub-markets such as medical
technology, diagnostics, curative health care pharmaceuticals,
hospital construction, ancillary services and curative health services. It is estimated to provide 81 per cent of outpatient care
and 46 per cent of inpatient care in India. Sixty-eight per cent
of India's 16,000 hospitals and 37 per cent of its 600,000 beds
are in the private sector.

The need for inpatient care is anticipated to rise sharply on
account of the increasing incidence of lifestyle diseases such as

cancer, Cardio Vascular Disease (CVD), diabetes, etc. To meet this rising demand for care, it has been estimated that an additional 750,000 beds, 520,000 doctors and an overall investment of Rupees 100–150 billion will be needed. Moreover, 80 per cent of this expenditure is projected to come from the private sector. Following the failures of public investments in health care and the process of liberalisation, several industrial/pharmaceutical companies and Non-Resident Indians (NRIs) are investing money in super-specialty hospitals such as, L.V. Prasad Eye Institute (Hyderabad), Max Health Care, Escorts Heart Institute and Research Centre (Delhi), P. D. Hindujas National Hospital and Research Centre and Wockhardt Heart Hospital (Mumbai).

PPP: Implications for primary health care

In 2004, eight median districts[1] were evaluated from the states of West Bengal, Maharashtra, Andhra Pradesh, Bihar, Uttar Pradesh, Madhya Pradesh and Rajasthan. The ratio of public-private facilities was found to be 60:40 in rural areas and 10:90 in urban areas. In the poorest blocks, the presence of the private sector was found to be negligible. Additionally, two thirds of health facilities and 79 per cent beds were found in urban areas, and 90 per cent of diagnostic equipment were concentrated in just a few limited urban centres.

A block has an average population of 100,000 people. Nearly 75 per cent of blocks surveyed have just three hospital beds, and there are examples of rural districts, such as 'Nadia' in West Bengal, that had a population of 190,000 and no hospital beds at all. Even though the government mandates that emergency obstetric facilities must exist in all blocks of India, the study found that 70 per cent of blocks had no emergency obstetric care facilities.

Overall, the private sector share in these eight districts was estimated as 52 per cent, which is lower than the 81 per cent estimate cited in the 52nd Round of National Sample Survey (NSS). It was found that bed occupancy for inpatient care was 44 per cent in private facilities and 62 per cent in the public sector. It should be noted, however, that this study of eight median districts confined itself to qualified providers, whereas NSS data may have covered unqualified providers as well.

An analysis of this study suggests a need to revise models for the location of primary health care facilities, as distribution of beds and specialists was highly skewed. Duplication of public and private facilities was found almost everywhere: private sector services are located precisely where public sector providers are already established. Thirty per cent of private hospitals employ government doctors to work in small rural nursing homes and city hospitals, which leads to significant 'conflict of interest' issues. The existence of multiple facilities in the same location within a small market area, that is, clustered near a Community Health Centre (CHC), may increase options for consumers. This may in turn promote two visible outcomes: first of all, it encourages un-ethical practises to cut costs among providers in order to maintain competitiveness; and second, it can lead to sub-optimal utilisation of public primary health care facilities and subsequently higher out-of-pocket (OOP) expenditure for the poorest households.

Non-alignment of facility locations with regard to demand tends to create problems. If there is an assured population base, whose health needs require care per provider then alternate payment systems like the capitation system of the National Health Scheme (UK) could be considered. This system requires the provider to be within close distance and accessible at all times. Right now, there may be an 'adequate' number of available qualified providers, but they need to be de-concentrated and re-distributed more equitably so that populations can be 'attached' to providers for basic health care. Public-Private Partnership design at primary health care levels should be based on a range of services rather than only on one-time activities such as delivery, immunisation, or sterilisation. As this will require a multi-skilled health team, the sole practitioner must accordingly expand his facility to conform to standards. To achieve this, it is necessary to perform detailed micro-planning of facilities that is guided by regulations, financial incentives and negotiation processes for re-distribution.

Kerala vs Bihar: A case study

The resulting policy package will stimulate re-organisation and re-structuring of the public and private sectors to allow more viable units and more equitable coverage that is in accordance with functional needs. The current literature on policy, programmes and primary health care in India iterates that the Central Government should cease spending money on health sub-centres in Kerala, as sound infrastructure like road connectivity already exists there. Money instead should be spent in poorer states like Bihar, as Bihar needs not only mobile hospitals but also mobile connectivity. Such spending discrepancies have resulted in a higher percentage of institutional deliveries in Kerala (99 per cent) as compared to Bihar. Additionally, as 275 per 100,000 persons die of CVD in Rajasthan compared to just 187 per 100,000 in Kerala, it could be said that possibly some of the deaths in Rajasthan could have been avoided with better access to timely treatment. Altogether, this implies that any solution must address real needs in the most problematic places. Additionally, the process should include a sustained dialogue on health insurance.

Against all drawbacks and from the standpoint of the government, the main task of PPPs is to ensure that people are not forced to shift to expensive private provision as a result of the public health sector's inefficiency. This is important because the private sector is exploitative and three to four times more expensive than the public sector. Typically, the poorest segments of society forgo health care entirely, except in life threatening situations, at which point they slide into severe debt. The 52nd Round of NSS showed that 35 per cent of the patients hospitalised in Bihar were pushed into severe debt resulting from medical expenditures, as compared to just 16 per cent in Kerala.

It is found that over 90 per cent of health care in Bihar is provided by the private sector, whereas only 60 per cent of care in Kerala is private. Over three-quarters of specialists and nearly 90 per cent of technology is in the private sector, concentrated in just a few towns. This divide must be bridged.

Need to prescribe standards and treatment protocols

Treatment costs across the private sector rise by about 20 per cent every year, and such growth is not sustainable for any government or insurance system. Therefore, it would be useful for the government to look at service unit costs to gain an understanding of the unreasonable private pricing structures. In doing so, cost benchmarks would be created that enable fair and rational judgement regarding the extent to which private pricing structures are unreasonable. This will also enable the government to enhance equity by re-directing higher investment into Primary Health Centres (PHCs) or city-based hospitals rather than continuing with health sub-centres.

Provider markets need to be restructured and health care providers must be re-deployed. There is no 'free' health care—someone must pay, either directly through user fees or indirectly through taxes.

Service delivery today is based on the discretionary judgement of the provider. The duality of protecting patient interests and accruing potential profit creates a grey area, with excess services such as irrational test/procedure prescription or unnecessarily long hospital stays occurring to generate more money. Such corruption can take many forms, however: doctors are found to own their own pharmacy shops; fee splitting occurs between diagnostic centres and referring doctors; and Ayurveda, Yoga and Naturopathy, Unani, Siddha and Homeopathy (AYUSH) doctors have been found prescribing allopathic drugs. To combat this, the government must prescribe and institutionalise standards and treatment protocols without delay. Such reforms would provide a basis for enforcing provider accountability, checking unethical practises and addressing conflict of interest issues.

Not-for-profit sector at primary health care levels

The government should look into the prospect of third sector involvement in primary health care as a credible alternative to the currently cash strapped, poorly managed public health system and expensive private system. If so, the government should provide financial and technical support to strengthen this sector's ability to offer reliable health care services, particularly in rural areas.

At the primary care level, the Non-Governmental Organisation (NGO) sector has some advantages over the private sector, as they can employ workers at lower wages in the form of contracts. NGOs can utilise specialist services on an honorary basis and can also use generic drugs and referrals. Additionally, this sector could have beneficial impacts on the accessibility, equity and quality of services in rural and backward areas. It indicates the possibility to mandate the third sector into the Public-Private Model.

Figure 4.1 Integration of the third sector into the PP model

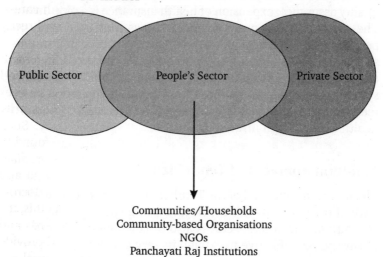

Communities/Households
Community-based Organisations
NGOs
Panchayati Raj Institutions

Therefore, direct investments towards the people's sector to build capacity will empower village health committees to exercise their Right to Information. In China, every village clinic displays the names and working hours of the doctors/nurses/traditional medicine practitioners and the listing of medicines/drugs assigned to the clinic. Such a system will also facilitate village and block health committees to do a social audit of the services and supplies mandated for the said village/block, in terms of nurses and doctors who were to attend work, or the medicines and drugs that were to reach the said village/block.

Quality of care

Public health goals are not properly integrated into either sector: the public sector is poorly funded, and private providers may seek to maximise profits through cost cutting, and both these factors result in low service quality. In Nigeria, the slogan 'free care is free death' highlights the 'care' found in the country's appalling public facilities. In order to motivate quality assurance systems, the government could examine the feasibility of capitation-based fees *in lieu* of service fees. Most important, however, is the recognition that without standards, treatment protocols and quality assurance, expansion of health insurance is a pipe dream. The current situation across India shows that even with the people's sector in the spotlight, we may not succeed in installing sustainable PPP interventions without the institution of standards, treatment protocols and quality assurance. Quality assurance systems can be motivated through systems for capitation-based fees, and this in turn will facilitate universal access to quality health care through insurance protocols.

Mid-term Appraisal of Tenth Plan

The mid-term appraisal of the Tenth plan recognised the import-ance of the government's involvement in quality assurance and regulation. The public sector is also discovering that it may not always be cost-effective to expand its services without engaging diverse sectors through multiple partnerships at different levels of care, including partnerships with the private sector. However, any such partnership between the public and private sectors must be mindful of potential repercussions on welfare such as in-creasing cost of health care. Thus, the inclusion of the people's sector is central to any PPP model. As government resources are limited and precious, their use should be limited to innovative financing strategies such as universal social insurance or subsidised community financing options for expansion of access to health care. The mid-term appraisal suggests that separate roles should be delineated for payer and provider, thereby facilitating health service contracts, strengthening accountability and empowering users in their relationships with providers. Rural, peri-urban and urban primary health facilities can be energised through franchised networks of diverse health providers across the civil society and the public and private sectors.

Initiatives at state government levels

In India, there are PPP initiatives at the state government level in three states: Arunachal Pradesh, Nagaland and Chhattisgarh. In Arunachal Pradesh, one PHC in each of the 16 districts was handed over to a reputed NGO, which was charged with providing clinical and public health services. It was anticipated that service delivery would be more predictable and would thus lead to higher utilisation of public facilities. This model was successful in Arunachal Pradesh.

In Nagaland, the village health committees took responsibility for maintaining health sub-centres, promoting public health interventions and also for popularising traditional systems of medicine. All the health sub-centres were communitised and thereby become a people's movement, resulting in lower absenteeism and improvements in staff salary disbursement and medicine availability.

In Chhattisgarh, there is a joint venture approach to high-end care. The state government has awarded Escorts Hospital a grant to build a state-of-the-art cardiology care hospital within the campus of the State Medical College. Pathology and laboratory tests are also sourced from the State Medical College. In Chhattisgarh, the Mitanin programme is run through a civil-state society programme that is fully aligned with health sector reform and as a result, increases the supply side of health care. Sixty thousand Mitanins have been recruited since 2002 in all 16 districts.

Anticipated outcomes of PPP

1. Cost effectiveness: The service provider is selected on the basis of pre-determined benchmarks and is contracted to provide reliable health services.
2. Higher productivity: Payments are linked to performance so that productivity increases.
3. Accelerated delivery of goods: Incentives and penalty clauses are written into contracts, as is an implementation process for these clauses.
4. Client focussed: Service is shifted to be output or outcome directed, thereby better addressing customer needs.

Distorted provider markets that have promoted an inequitable, inefficient and expensive system must be regulated and corrected. The private sector has invested a significant amount of resources and the government need not duplicate these investments, but should rather attempt to direct resources towards achieving public health goals. This is possible only with dialogue between the two sectors. Any new investment must be need-based and include the people's sector so that the investments maintain focus on social safety nets while ensuring successful development of PPP.

Apart from the needed consensus among professional organisations and consumer advocacy forums, quality assurance mechanisms, comprehensive regulation and standard treatment protocols are also necessary for better implementation of public-private partnerships.

Note

1. Identified through the Centre for Monitoring Indian Economy (CMIE) index, 1991.

Private-Public Participation in the Control of Tuberculosis in Tamil Nadu and Kerala (India): What is its Future?

5

V.R. MURALEEDHARAN, SONIA ANDREWS, BHUVANESWARI R. AND STEPHEN JAN

Introduction

Public-private partnership (PPP) is a system in which a government service or private business venture is funded and operated through a partnership of government and one or more private sector companies. These schemes are sometimes referred to as PPP or 3-Ps. The developmental triangle described in Figure 5.1 by Dr Sen explains development in terms of 'real sharing', where different stakeholders divide responsibility to achieve better results (Sen 2000).

During the last decade in India, the concept of PPP gained much prominence in the health care sector. The foremost objective of such partnerships is to improve the 'accessibility and quality' of health care at relatively lower costs. In order to control the spread of Tuberculosis (TB), the World Health Organisation (WHO) has promoted the strategy of Directly Observed Treatment, Short course (DOTS). The Revised National Tuberculosis Control Programme (RNTCP), which has adopted this strategy in India since early 1990s, has designed specific 'schemes' to involve Private Practitioners (PPs) and Non-Governmental Organisations (NGOs) in DOTS implementation throughout the country.

Figure 5.1 Development triangle in creating public-private partnership

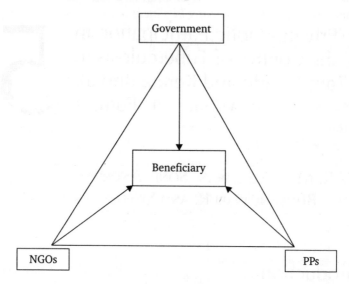

Components of RNTCP

The PPP schemes under RNTCP involve NGOs and PPs in some or all components, which consist of: (*i*) Health Education and Community Outreach; (*ii*) Provision of Directly Observed Therapy; (*iii*) In-Hospital Care for Tuberculosis Disease; (*iv*) Diagnosis and Treatment; and (*v*) Referral. The effort of PPP has been a bottom-up approach in India. This movement started at the grassroots level and expanded its focus upwards, with the acceptance of the PPP concept by the government machinery happening over the years. With the increasing success of PPP, it is now important to expand PPP's radius to address policy issues.

The Revised National Tuberculosis Control Programme has been a pioneer in this movement. There are specific schemes for involving NGOs and PPs in implementing RNTCP. Specific systems that involve NGO participation are health education and community outreach, provision of directly observed treatment, in-hospital care for TB, microscopy and treatment centres, TB unit models (which encompasses all of the above components) and lastly, plans for encouraging community involvement. On the other hand, schemes involving PPs include referral of suspected TB patients, provision of treatment observation and designated microscopy centres for microscopy only and for both microscopy and treatment.

Research questions

In the light of emerging policy foci, a study conducted from November 2003 through July 2004 in Tamil Nadu (TN) and Kerala examined the three fundamental policy questions:

1. Why should the private sector and NGOs be involved in the implementation of the RNTCP?
2. What has been the experience of the PPP strategy in implementing RNTCP?
3. What policy changes are required to strengthen PPP as a strategy in implementing RNTCP?

Methodology

The study adopted the method of triangulation, studying both qualitative and quantitative methods of data collection. It involved several field visits (in nine districts of TN and Kerala) and interviews with more than 400 key informants, including 118 TB patients treated under RNTCP/DOTS. Specific Survey Instruments were developed for data collection from stakeholders, who included state officials, district TB officers such as State Tuberculosis Officer (STO), District Tuberculosis Officer (DTO), Medical Officer TB (MO-TB), NGOs, independent PPs, private hospitals, private microscopy centres, community volunteers working as DOTS providers, field workers such as Village Health Nurses (VHNs), private funding agencies (supporting NGOs/hospitals), state-level policy-cont officials and patients. The interviews were conducted from four districts in Kerala and five districts in TN, covering more than 20 Tuberculosis Units (TUs) in all. Each TU covers a population of five hundred thousand.

Understanding the present structure of PPPs, a key question must be asked regarding existing schemes: What is the best way to involve NGOs and PPs in fulfilling the objectives of RNTCP?

Analysis

Any change draws resistance, and the test of time is the best method for determining whether outcomes of a new method are positive or negative. At the inception of PPP, research suggests both positive and negative impacts from this approach.

Rationale for adopting PPP

There are three key arguments for adopting PPP that address 'cost-effectiveness' of the RNTCP-treatment/drug regime. The first is that by converting PPs into the RNTCP-treatment regime, it is possible to reduce unnecessary drug consumption by patients. Second, it is argued that PPP would help in reducing 'barriers to access to care', as government infrastructure alone cannot possibly deliver care to every TB patient in India. The last argument contends that PPP will substantially reduce the 'financial burden' on the poor, since diagnostics, treatment and care would be provided free of cost under RNTCP.

Weaknesses affecting PPP

Overall participation of NGOs has been very limited in both TN and Kerala. As in most collaborations, both of these states are vested only with the responsibility of DOTS provision. However, in Kerala, many PPs are also involved with microscopy activities. Issues related to contractual arrangements, lack of personnel for DOTS supervision, financial aid and practise of 'dual treatment regimes' are some of the major factors that influence implementation of PPP schemes. There are numerous possibilities for strengthening the PPP strategy. Future policy measures should aim to: (*i*) encourage private practitioners to accept the treatment regimes prescribed by RNTCP through better information and training; (*ii*) involve NGOs and PPs to a greater extent via better incentive mechanisms; and (*iii*) increase manpower to better monitor and supervise the NGOs/PPs involved in RNTCP.

Challenges and constraints in implementing PPP

There are some constraints and challenges of PPP implementation under RNTCP that must be addressed. One of the most important issues concerns contractual arrangements, whereby NGOs and PPs are involved only on an 'informal' basis in implementation of PPP schemes. Also, it has been observed that direct observation of patients by DOT providers is lower than 50 per cent. Most PPs have 'dual treatment regimes', with separate regimes for the poor to whom RNTCP drugs are given, and another for 'those with money', who then buy drugs from the market. As a senior chest physician from Kerala said:

> I have two lists of patients. One consists of those put under the DOTS regime. These are either referred to us by nearby government health centres or are poor patients who cannot afford to buy drugs on their own. The second list consists of professionals (such as lawyers, engineers) who can afford to buy medicines on their own. These patients also do not wish to be supervised frequently and therefore do not wish to be on DOTS regime.

Again, most PPs and NGOs do not have any field staff dedicated to DOTS implementation. However, most NGOs and PPs (both in TN and Kerala) were not aware of the different design features of schemes in which they were involved. Many NGOs also reported considerable delay in receiving annual grant approval from various proposals, while some of them did not receive any endorsement beyond staff salary and travel. In TN, NGOs and PPs do not pay financial incentives to volunteers, whereas in Kerala, most volunteers are paid financial incentives. Supervisory staff experience several logistical and operational difficulties in supervising DOTS providers due to its geographic coverage.

There are diverse views within the government bureaucracy regarding the desirability of involving the private sector. Several key government officials do not believe, for ideological or other practical reasons, that the private sector should play any role in the health sector. There has also been an overall lack of training of PPs in RNTCP.

Different challenges to PPP implementation of RNTCP-based schemes exist, such as lack of belief in efficacy of RNTCP regimes, fear of patient loss and subsequent loss of income, reluctance to deal with bureaucracy, lack of awareness of PPP programmes, and lack of support of all officials for PPP. As a chest physician from a government hospital in TN said:

> We are not allowed to prescribe any regime that is different from that of RNTCP, although my experience in the past 15 years has been that it is inadequate. I wear two hats always: I prescribe the RNTCP regime for patients admitted into government hospital where I work, whereas I prescribe quite another regime for patients I examine in my private practice. I firmly believe in the latter, but I cannot say this in the presence of my state officials because I am "supposed" to believe in the national regime of the RNTCP.

Policy lessons learnt

Sustained experimentation with PPP requires overarching policy support. This not only calls for legislative support of PPP, but also for a larger debate that will facilitate consensus and cooperation. At present, PPP is seen as an immediate solution for overcoming existing weaknesses in the delivery system, but it is ultimately driven largely by the likes and dislikes of programme managers. This model is not an end in itself, but instead requires building credibility into the public health care system and policy-making machinery through careful understanding of the political economy of statistics.

Counter argument

Even after targets are achieved, it is necessary to continue PPP, as measures are often manipulated once they become part of targets. In the light of this, two informative quotations come to mind: a Chinese proverb, 'Officials make the figures and the figures make the officials', and Goodhart's Law, which states that an 'indicator's measurement will be distorted if it is used as a target'.

Key policy suggestions

At present, as part of PPP strategy under RNTCP, there are more NGOs in urban areas than in rural areas. But there should be greater effort to involve NGOs in rural areas. Efforts should be made to engage NGOs working in sectors other than health (such as education, environment and micro-credit financing) as DOTS providers and in implementing Information, Education and Communication (IEC) campaigns. 'Informal' contractual arrangements are common and are currently seen as the preferred method by many stakeholders. Therefore, it is important to formalise all partnerships, as doing so encourages better monitoring and commitment from all stakeholders involved.

Programme managers must ensure that grant-in-aid and incentives are sanctioned and released on time to partners, as per contracts, in order to sustain continuity in service provision. The current schemes for involving NGOs/PPs require considerable modification. For example, several PPs do not find incentives under the present PPP schemes attractive enough. It is thus necessary to evolve a uniform structure of financial incentives for DOTS providers under PPP schemes. At present, very few Self Help Group (SHG) members are engaged as DOTS providers and therefore, efforts should be made to involve them across regions, as SHGs operate in several parts of the country. As most NGOs and PPs do not have adequate field staff for DOTS supervision, RNTCP should provide more support for the hiring of field staff, particularly to NGOs in hilly regions, for supervisory role improvement.

There is a need to address RNTCP training for laboratory technicians and medical officers in NGOs and PPs. Many NGOs and PPs have infrequent interaction with programme officials, and most have also not participated in periodic review meetings conducted by officials. Programme managers should make greater efforts to involve NGOs/PPs in the planning process.

Regular inspection and servicing of equipment (such as micro-scopes) supplied by RNTCP to NGOs should be carried out to improve their performance. Questions regarding the extent to which private practitioners must be convinced of the RNTCP treatment regime's efficacy must be answered. Evidence from our study shows that very few PPs believe in and practise the DOTS regime prescribed by RNTCP. Related to this, another challenge to implementation of the RNTCP-based PPP strategy lies in investigating the beliefs of public sector physicians in practis-ing the RNTCP prescribed drug-protocol, as they are currently unknown. The progress and impact of PPP strategy suffers from many bureaucratic pulls and pressures, but this may be true for several developmental programmes, particularly in the health sector and with respect to RNTCP. The attitude of government officials towards NGOs/PPs varies substantially across districts despite overarching policy-level support for the PPP strategy. However, this policy-level support does not identify any defini-tive 'legislative authority' that would compel the bureaucracy or programme managers to implement the PPP strategy more vigorously. It is difficult to visualise successful implementation of the PPP strategy in the coming years without greater political and bureaucratic commitment to transparency of the overall PPP strategy. Finally, it can be said that future success of the PPP strategy in implementation of RNTCP depends, to a great extent, on careful nurturing of the NGOs and community volunteers com-mitted to the promotion of public health.

Conclusion

A policy model cannot be implemented in isolation. After pilot-testing the three-fold PPP model in the health care sector (in two states of India under the TB programme) and analysing the research findings, it can be concluded that support is not only encouraged, but necessary, from other stakeholders in the public sector, private sector and from community organisations.

Reference

Sen, A.K. 2000. *Development as Freedom*. New Delhi: Oxford University Press.

Public-Private Partnership— Sri Lankan Experience

6

ARUNA RABEL

Introduction to public-private partnership in Sri Lanka

Traditionally, there has been an assumption that the state should directly manage health care facilities. However, in most developing countries, there has been some sort of private sector involvement as successive governments fail to improve their investments in the health sector and to provide services according to the expectations of all segments of the society. These countries consequently experience huge gaps between the demand and supply of health care, with the end result being an ever-increasing burden of health care expenses placed directly on families. In developing countries, a strong though informal network of 'Traditional Health Care Providers' prevails for several obvious reasons.

Sri Lanka, a smaller and comparatively lesser developed nation than India, has a better-managed health care service delivery system. Through the last two decades, Sri Lanka has constantly maintained 3.5 per cent of its GDP as the National Health Expenditure (NHE), with a per capita expenditure of 15 US dollars. More than 50 per cent of NHE is from private sources, with the remaining half coming from public sources. Household expenditure remains as high as 43 per cent of NHE. Though per capita expenditure on health in the country is quite low, a significant portion of the NHE is allocated to maintaining its 40,000-strong health care work force.

Figure 6.1 reflects the gradual decrease in public sector expenditure for health care in Sri Lanka. In 1990, the public and private expenditures in health care were almost the same, with a subsequent steady decrease in public sector expenditure till 1996. During 1999, with the partnership of the private sector, the government managed to increase expenditure in public health care.

Figure 6.1   Health expenditure in Sri Lanka as a percentage share of GDP

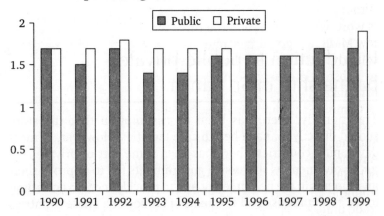

Sri Lanka's achievements in certain health indicators are quite impressive. The Maternal Mortality Rate (MMR) remains as low as 23 per 100,000 live births, Infant Mortality Rate (IMR) is 16.3 per 1,000 live births, and the neonatal mortality rate is 12.9 per 1,000 live births. The life expectancy of Sri Lankan women is 75 years, while it is 71 years for men. These figures speak highly of Sri Lanka and its effective primary health care management. The well-structured primary health care network and a high adult literacy rate (90.1 per cent) are identified as major contributing factors to this phenomenon. Nevertheless, due to several other priorities, which include national security, the state has found it difficult to invest in improving tertiary health care facilities such as cardiac surgery or advanced cancer therapy. This is a great disadvantage to the country, as funding organisations are unwilling to fund such advanced health programmes. But the private sector has come forward to invest in providing advanced tertiary health care facilities and continues to improve its investments. It has clearly emerged that close partnership between the public and private sectors must develop for the delivery of quality health care on a long term basis.

Sri Lanka is one of the most progressive models of Public-Private Partnership (PPP) and can be taken as a unique example for other developing countries. Since Independence in 1948, development indicators had risen in Sri Lanka until recently, when a stagnation was witnessed during the past five or six years. Although this chapter does not focus on maternal mortality, it is worthwhile to mention the three main factors for Sri Lanka's low MMR: a high literacy rate, unprecedented service delivered by midwives and steady health expenditure. These features help to substantiate arguments regarding the success of PPPs in Sri Lanka.

Common assumptions about PPPs are that health care must be provided by the state, that the private sector is only for the rich and that the private sector should not be involved with the state. Any move by the successive governments to improve the delivery of health care through a partnership has encountered resistance from the public and mainly from health care workers and their trade unions. Many such plans have been withdrawn and could never be implemented.

History of public-private partnership

Sri Lanka has many traditional systems of medicine that are closely tied to the state system. A strong institutional referral system exists, as does channel practise, due to a lack of available consultants in the private sector and as a means of avoiding 'brain drain' from Sri Lanka. Subsequent to the introduction of open economic policies in 1977, the state sector doctors were allowed to involve themselves in private practise. Specialists' channel practise thus began to receive a huge demand, particularly in areas where larger state hospitals were in operation. Patients began to enjoy the liberty of meeting the specialists as they wished, of course at an out-of-pocket cost.

Unofficial partnership

Another issue worth considering is unofficial partnership. Though official permission is given to medical professionals to engage in private consultations beyond working hours, often no official arrangement exists for them, thereby raising many ethical issues. Some controversial practises exist such as public servants having the opportunity to do private practise after working hours though many other professionals are not allowed to do so; private practitioners referring their cases to the state sector for secondary and tertiary management; and investigations or admissions through channel consultations leading to cases sent to the private sector, where the patient bears the cost of care.

Official partnership

Laboratory and other diagnostic services in the state sector hospitals are often disturbed due to trade union actions and breakdowns. The monopoly of the state over drug purchases was removed with the implementation of an open economy in 1977 and equipment purchases are done mainly through the private sector. The President's Fund provides assistance for major surgical procedures and certain tertiary level treatment received in the private sector as well as abroad. Apart from this, partnerships like the Employees' Trust Fund, the Social Services Ministry and the Government Servants' Insurance contribute immensely for people to receive health care from the private sector.

State policy

As per the 1996 National Health Policy, the government facilitates development and regulation of the private health care sector while promoting better coordination with it. After a decade of progress, current concerns are political interference, trade unions with vested interests, fear of 'privatisation', a lack of political commitment, absence of proper authority for coordination, poor awareness and absence of a legal framework that enables solutions for progressive systemic change.

Some results of poorly executed private-public partnerships are listed below:

1. Inefficient utilisation of available resources.
2. Unnecessary investment by both sectors.
3. Increased cost of health care.
4. Obstacles to quality assurance.
5. Inadequately planned health care delivery.

Investigations and admissions following channel consultations

Private practitioners refer their cases to the public sector for secondary and tertiary management, using the right of any citizen to receive free treatment from government hospitals. Poor people do utilise this opportunity as a sort of passport to gain certain privileges in government hospitals. When a patient meets a government consultant, he/she is given an admission note to enter a government hospital. These patients are then sent for further consultation or treatment, resulting in private patients being investigated at the cost of the state, though sometimes the patient bears a portion of the cost as well.

Purchase of drugs

This official partnership did not exist until open economic policies were introduced in Sri Lanka. Since opening the economy, the private sector has become equally involved in purchasing drugs as well as equipment, while the state just acts as a facilitator.

Further funding

In Sri Lanka, a lottery is drawn weekly that is marketed throughout the country and the revenue is diverted for further development of the state sector health care. The President's Fund receives contributions through another lottery and is also funded by many donor agencies and the fund spends a significant portion for the improvement of state sector health care institutions as well as for assisting individuals to receive tertiary level treatment in the private sector. However, there are duplicities and over-expenditure due to lack of public-private dialogue.

Trade unions

Trade unions are quite active in Sri Lanka's health sector. Trade union actions are common ranging from work to rule campaigns to general strikes, mainly on policy matters. Whenever the diagnostic services are affected by trade union actions, state hospitals are compelled to call for assistance from private sector in order to maintain at least basic patient care services.

Whenever there is no existing partnership, it becomes impossible for either sector to deliver services effectively. Some advantages of participatory planning include multi-sectoral collaboration, reduction in costs, increased efficiency of health care, a decreased service gap, resource sharing, better quality assurance, improved community participation and greater donor agency confidence. However, there are many places where quality health care does not extend to poorer segments of the society. Some areas for partnership are primary and secondary health care, with a special focus on tertiary care.

Conclusion

In the light of the discussion, it can be concluded that training of health care personnel and health care planning are the two main areas that demand PPP to better the delivery of services and management of health care. A public-private dialogue must be initiated by the government to begin the journey of participation. Sri Lanka's radical approach in practising a partnership model for health care has expanded the reach of its health network, benefiting health sector professionals as well as the people of the country. This innovative model could and should be replicated in other densely populated, under-resourced developing countries so that the civil right of 'good health for all citizens of the world' can be achieved.

Governance in Health Systems 7

S.R. RAO

The Constitution of India envisages the establishment of a new social model based on equality, freedom, justice and dignity of the individual. It aims for elimination of poverty and of ignorance towards health and thereby seeks to raise the level of nutrition and the standard of living of its citizens. It emphasises that better public health is every state's primary objective, placing priority on the health and strength of its people, especially on ensuring the growth of children in a healthy environment. The approaches of previous planning documents may have generally served the needs of some, but there is still a need to develop a comprehensive approach towards the progress of medical education, research and health services in order to serve the actual health needs and priorities of all people.

In spite of some progress, the demographic and health pictures of India are still cause for serious concern. The high and distressing rate of population growth, maternal and child mortality, severity of malnutrition, the emerging challenge of non-communicable diseases, lack of basic sanitation, etc., mandate that it is time to reformulate the vision and mission of our health care system. Without community involvement, the ultimate goal of a satisfactory health status cannot be achieved. Thus, it is necessary to identify a community's health needs and priorities for the management of various health related programmes.

This chapter emphasises the involvement of the private sector in meeting the demands of the health care sector in the state of Gujarat in order to reach the masses better. Ensuring health service at an affordable cost is another issue of concern. However, the real challenge is to expand the corollaries of the 'multiplier effect' by extending services to the rural areas. The government has been quite successful in acknowledging the model of 'multiplier effect' and has subsequently developed a 'three tier system' of management. Medicine has been one of the most progressive sectors in India, but the reach of health care has lagged behind. Many issues of concern in Western countries, such as availability of counsellors in schools or hospitals, have not received any recognition in our country.

The LaLonde Model: The LaLonde model was first proposed by LaLonde in 1974, with a focus on health promotion. Later, in the year 2003, it was expanded to include 12 determinants. The determinants of health mentioned in the model are: (*i*) income and social status; (*ii*) social support networks; (*iii*) education and literacy; (*iv*) employment and working conditions; (*v*) social environments; (*vi*) physical environments; (*vii*) personal health practise and coping skills; (*viii*) healthy child development; (*ix*) biology and genetic endowment; (*x*) health services (access to health care); (*xi*) gender; and (*xii*) culture (*Population Health*, Thomas University).

One of the main outcomes of the LaLonde model was an increased focus on individual lifestyle changes. Disability, disease and death are the main aspects of health and thus, well-being can be seen as a result of the complex interplay of various determinants. The cause and effect of these aspects can be modified to various degrees by health protection, prevention and promotion, or by treatment and rehabilitation. Such interventions need support from human and material resources, including essential information obtained through research, monitoring and evaluation (European Commission).

The LaLonde Model has become the cornerstone of all preventive policy. It distinguishes the many different aspects of health, which are determined by four factors: heredity, environment, lifestyle and health care (see Figure 7.1).

During the last decade, a remarkable change has occurred in medical science: the gap between knowledge and technology has narrowed, as seen by the use of outstanding skill in intensive care to save many lives. However, at the national level the goals of many public health interventions could not be achieved,

Figure 7.1   Inputs to Health—LaLonde Model

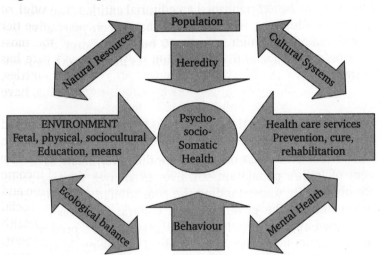

leaving the nation with an overwhelming unfinished agenda. On comparing the demographic situations of India and China, it is evident that India, while being a less populated country, has a comparatively low female literacy rate and life expectancy (see Table 7.1).

Empirical data shows that chronic diseases or 'lifestyle diseases' grow alongside economic growth. Modern medicine has been successful in finding cures for diseases such as polio and smallpox, but at the present level of communication, medicine's

Table 7.1   Demographic situation of China and India

Indicators	China	India
Population (in million)	1288	1064
Life expectancy (in years)	71	63
Female adult literacy (percentage)	87	45
Under-five mortality (per 1,000 children)	37	87
Under-five malnutrition (percentage)	12	45

Source: UNDP, Human Development Report 2006. *Beyond Scarcity: Power, Poverty and the Global Water Crisis.* New York: Palgrave MacMillan.

access to public health is limited. In its special edition on child survival, *The Lancet* published an editorial entitled 'The World's Forgotten Children', which showed that fifteen years after the world summit on children, over 10 million children die every year before the age of five due to failures in the health delivery system.

Governance in health systems

Public health is a cause of concern for the government, as 60 per cent of India's population still lives in villages with agrarian livelihoods. By understanding the core strength of community interventions, the government of Gujarat recognises that a 'top-down approach' will not be successful in the present situation. Communities should be involved in making decisions regarding health delivery systems, and as NGOs are community based organisations, they could prove to be a strong medium in achieving this goal. Over the past several years, through NGOs, national health services have established links to local communities who manage these hospitals. Along with this, there are various issues to take into consideration, such as human resources, financing, legal frameworks, personnel management, supplies and equipment, nutrition (improved and scientific utilisation of available food material, prevention of food adulteration), maintenance of drug quality, water supply and sanitation, environmental protection, school health and occupational health services.

There are 38,000 health personnel, 6,500 qualified doctors and 3,000 trainers in the Indian system of medicine. Similarly, there are close to 10,000 other staff and field workers in the health sector. The government has 122 different types of designations, some in use since the British time, including the post of thermometer washer (whose only duty was to wash thermometers), which was discontinued only recently. As compared to the other states of India, the Government of Gujarat's expenditure on health care is quite high. Even though there are an adequate number of machines in the hospitals (district hospitals have four x-ray machines), including standbys, machine maintenance is mainly neglected.

The government's strength has to be used by hospital boards to ensure transparency, accountability and performance improvement. This is done by taking proper steps, which involve strategic planning, monitoring of organisational performance, clinical quality assurance, patient safety, annual budgeting, creation of a positive employee culture, medical staff relations, policy lobbying of government and finally, reporting performance to public.

Public-private partnership

Due to moral vulnerabilities of the medical staff, private practise is not allowed in the government sector. However, in tribal and border areas where medical facilities are not available, collaboration with the private sector is encouraged. After analysing the situation in slums over several years, it was observed that people living in slum areas spend much more on water and hospitals as compared to the middle class. People must stand in a queue when they visit the public hospital, and as hospital visits are often time away from work, people lose wages while waiting. As a result, they prefer to opt for private services and pay out of pocket. Concerns regarding housing, water and health include quality and accessibility. In the current situation, if the government assures service, people will pay for them, as they do not need subsidised health care services.

Public-private partnership should incorporate District Rural Health Missions, District Health Societies and the emergency medical services scheme. Primary Health Centres (PHCs) and Community Health Centres (CHCs) should be handed over to Trust Managed Organisations/Voluntary Organisations (NGOs) for optimal productivity. Consideration should also be given to large district hospitals for establishment of tertiary cardiac care centres. Zilla Rogi Kalyan Samitis must be established for patient welfare activities.

There is a need to provide primary health care, placing special emphasis on the preventive, promotional and rehabilitative aspects. Approaches for restructuring health services should provide a well-dispersed network of primary health services while integrating non-governmental organisations and private institutions within a time-bound programme and by also training health volunteers in simple skills and technologies. Other approaches of reform are well-furnished referral systems and packages of services to overcome poor health conditions. Establishing low-cost curative centres with all modern equipment and offering organised logistical, financial and technical support to voluntary health agencies will also be helpful. This, in turn, can encourage individual self-reliance and community participation with the support of secondary and tertiary levels of health care services. The organisation of programmes for sectors of mental health and for the medical care and rehabilitation of mentally retarded, deaf, dumb, blind, physically disabled, infirm and elderly populations are other issues that need to be addressed.

Under the concept of re-orientation, a dynamic process of change and innovation should be used for the whole approach of promoting the concept of 'Health Team' that is, the vast untapped resources of AYUSH practioners should be integrated and health education programmes should be nationally supported by appropriate communication strategies. Even after extensive progress in Gujarat, only 10 million school children are covered by the network of government and voluntary private doctors.

An effective health information system is required for planning, decision-making, forecasting, reviewing and monitoring of the programmes. Along with this, there is a need for innovation of sound technological and manufacturing capability in the fields of drugs, vaccines, biomedical equipment etc., especially for emerging challenges like HIV. Health insurance is necessary for mobilising additional resources and for ensuring that the community shares the cost of services. Health and human development must ultimately constitute an integral component of the overall socioeconomic development process in the country.

Medical audits and evaluation of the quality of the medical care provided by physicians should be undertaken to detect deficiencies and ensure collective accountability for quality care. In a couple of districts in Gujarat, tele-medicine and Management Information Systems (MIS) for the health sector, which can be used as early detection systems for epidemics, are under trial.

These systems have also been extended to other departments and commercial auditing is being conducted by professional Chartered Accountants (CAs). It is clear that there are ample resources, but there is a need to overcome coordination deficits and to concurrently strengthen the traditional Indian system of medicine. Every year, there are new problems and therefore new, creative solutions must be developed for these problems. Finally, it can be said that

> We may have missed in achieving 'Health For All by 2000 AD' but let us strive to make 'Vision 2020' a reality. We have most likely failed due to poverty-of-vision and not as a result of poverty-of-funds. No matter how bleak the situation is, there are always alternatives (Polish Proverb).

References

European Commission. 2004. 'Building a European System of Information and Knowledge on Major and Chronic Diseases, Version 3. EC,' Health & Consumer Protection Directorate-General. Working Party Morbidity and Mortality, Task Force Major and Chronic Diseases, Task Force on Rare Diseases. Luxembourg, 12–14 October. Available online at http://ec.europa.eu/health/ph_information/implement/wp/morbidity/docs/ev_20041012_co01_en.pdf (Accessed on 12 September 2007).

National Conference of Indian Academy of Pediatrics. 2005. 'Presidential Address, XXXXII', *Indian Pediatrics* 117(42), 17 February.

The Lancet Editorial. 2003. 'The World's Forgotten Children', *The Lancet*, 361(9351): 1.

Thomas University. 'Population Health', an online course for public health professionals, Unit 1, Module 1, available online at http://www.thomasu.edu/people/Mdolen/html/u1module1.htm).

UNDP Human Development Report. 2006. *Beyond Scarcity: Power, Poverty and the Global Water Crisis*. New York: Palgrave MacMillan.

Good Governance in Health Services

8

H. SUDARSHAN

Good governance is one of the most important factors in improving health services. Merely adding new technological packages is not enough and they may improve the outcome marginally. Through good governance we can achieve a quantum jump in health outcomes.

Transparency International (TI) has been bringing out a Corruption Perception Index (CPI) every year. Transparency International-India did an empirical survey with the help of Org-Marg Private Ltd in 2004. The study clearly shows the health sector as the most corrupt, following the police. A similar study during 2005 also shows that government hospitals are the most corrupt amongst the five public sectors which provide basic needs—schools, water supply, PDS, electricity and government hospitals.

The report of the Task Force on Health and Family Welfare, Government of Karnataka, under the chairmanship of Dr H. Sudarshan, has also put Corruption in health services at the top of the list of 'Major issues of Concern'. The Karnataka Lokayuktha, an ombudsman organisation at the state level, has also data to show that health sector is one of the most corrupt sectors. The corruption in public health services has become an epidemic. We need to study and understand the pathogenesis, the aetiological factors, diagnosis and management of this epidemic. The eradication or elimination of corruption may be a distant dream. But we can certainly control it.

Effective management and supervision, e-governance for transparency and accountability, training in Health Management for doctors, hospital committees, citizen's charter, report card system, strengthening the consumer forum, and awareness about Right to Information Act and Transparency Act are some of the measures which can bring good governance in health services.

The proactive Karnataka Lokayukta headed by retired Supreme Court Justice N. Venkatachala and assisted by Dr H. Sudarshan, Vigilance Director, has made substantial progress in improving governance in Public Health Services in Karnataka.

Introduction

New technological innovations are not enough to improve health outcomes—good governance is also necessary for progress in health services. Through good governance, a quantum jump in health care outcomes can be achieved. Corruption is rampant in India. Every year, TI comes out with the CPI, ranking various countries around the world. More than two-thirds of the 158 nations surveyed under the 2005 TI-CPI scored less than five out of an optimal clean score of 10, indicating serious levels of corruption in their system. The CPI for India was 2.9, with a worldwide rank of 88. Iceland had the lowest level of corruption, while Bangladesh and Chad were found to be the most corrupt countries (see Table 8.1).

Transparency International-Corruption Perception Index projected corruption levels among Indian states during 2005 through an empirical survey with ORG-Marg Private Ltd. Bihar was determined to be the most corrupt state in India, whereas Kerala was the least corrupt (see Table 8.2).

This study covered 10 sectors, which included the police, health, education, Public Distribution System (PDS), land administration, judiciary, taxation, railways and telecom departments. Among need-based services, the police department was the most corrupt in the Indian government whereas the telecom department was the least (see Table 8.3). However, in basic services, the government hospitals were the most corrupt. Regional distribution of the Indian CPI shows that the health department attained the highest score in eastern India, whereas in the north,

**Table 8.1   Transparency International Corruption
Perceptions Index**

Year	Score for India	Rank of India	Countries with lowest level of corruption	Countries with highest level of corruption
1995	2.78	34/41	New Zealand	Indonesia
1996	2.63	45/54	New Zealand	Nigeria
1997	2.75	44/54	Denmark	Nigeria
1998	2.90	66/85	Denmark	Cameroon
1999	2.90	72/99	Sweden	Cameroon
2000	2.80	69/90	Finland	Nigeria
2001	2.70	71/91	Finland	Bangladesh
2002	2.70	71/102	Finland	Bangladesh
2003	2.80	83/133	Finland	Bangladesh
2004	2.80	90/145	Finland	Bangladesh & Haiti
2005	2.90	88/158	Iceland	Bangladesh & Chad

Source: Transparency International Corruption Perceptions Index, 1995–2005.

**Table 8.2   Corruption Study of India by Transparency
International India, 2005**

State	C. Index	Rank	State	C. Index	Rank
Kerala	240	1	Delhi	496	11
Himachal Pradesh	301	2	Tamil Nadu	509	12
Gujarat	417	3	Haryana	516	13
Andhra Pradesh	433	4	Jharkhand	520	14
Maharashtra	433	5	Assam	542	15
Chhattisgarh	445	6	Rajasthan	543	16
Punjab	459	7	Karnataka	576	17
West Bengal	461	8	M.P.	584	18
Orissa	475	9	J & K	655	19
Uttar Pradesh	491	10	Bihar	695	20

Source: Transparency International India, India Corruption Study, 2005.

south and west, the police department was the most corrupt. This data also indicates that the health and power sectors are those with the most impact on society, making them highly corruptible departments.

Table 8.3   Corruption index and ranking of services

Need-based Services			Basic Services		
	C. Index	Rank		C. Index	Rank
Rural Financial Institutions	22	1	Schools	26	1
Income Tax	35	2	Water Supply	29	2
Municipalities	47	3	PDS	37	3
Judiciary	59	4	Electricity	39	4
Land Admin	59	5	Govt. Hospitals	42	5
Police	77	6			

Source: Transparency International India, India Corruption Study, 2005.

The epidemic of corruption in health services at the national level

The basic services are government monopolies. It is clear that the health sector, specifically government hospitals, is perceived to be the most corrupt sector in basic service while also having the highest public interaction (8 per cent) and greatest societal impact, affecting a population of 81 crore people. Health comprises nearly the highest portion of the bribe amount paid, at 40 per cent (Rs 75.7 billion) of the total (Rs 267 billion) (Transparency International India 2005). Bribe payment is typically done through hospital staff, and demand for money is more common in southern India (38 per cent) than northern (25 per cent). Even amongst the medical staff, it was widely felt that doctors demanded more than the other staff.

Task force on department of health and family welfare, Government of Karnataka

Corruption in public health services has become an epidemic. It is now necessary to study and understand the etiology and pathogenesis of this epidemic so as to develop a diagnosis and for proper management of this 'disease'. Although it may not be possible to 'eradicate' corruption like small pox, it can indeed be 'controlled', like tuberculosis. The Government of Karnataka constituted a Task Force on Health and Family Welfare under my chairmanship (*vide* Government Order No. HFW 545 CGM 99) on 14 December 1999. The mission of the Task Force was to make recommendations for improvements in public health and on major issues like population stabilisation, departmental management and administration, educational system reform covering both clinical and public health sectors, and developing a plan for monitoring the implementation of these recommendations.

The final report of the Task Force highlighted 12 major issues concerning health care and placed corruption right on the top. The other 11 issues were neglect of public health, distortions in primary health care, lack of focus on equity, gaps in implementation, neglect of ethics and law, neglect of human resource development, cultural gap and medical pluralism, from exclusivism to partnership, ignoring the political economy of health, neglect of research, and countering the growing apathy in the system. The Task Force concluded that corruption in health services is the major issue of concern, even in Karnataka.

History of Karnataka Lokayukta

The present Karnataka Lokayukta had its beginnings in the Mysore State Vigilance Commission established in 1965. In 1984, the Karnataka Lokayukta Act came into existence and the Karnataka Lokayukta Rules were set the following year. In September of 1986, the Karnataka Lokayukta Act was amended and *suo moto* prosecution powers against officials with a basic salary above Rs 10,600 per month was withdrawn, thus removing all the senior officers, bureaucrats and ministers from the purview of the Lokayukta. However, there is still a provision of proceeding against any government servant on the basis of a complaint with an affidavit. The Act authorises investigation of any government servant, encompassing the chief minister; ministers and all members of the state legislature; any officer of the state government; the chair, vice-chair, and any person employed by local authorities and corporations; any registered society or co-operative society; and any university established by or under any law of the legislature. The cause of the Lokayukta was further strengthened with the inclusion of the Prevention of Corruption Act in 1988.

The Karnataka Lokayukta has four wings: the police wing to execute traps and raids, the judiciary wing to manage complaints and reports, technical wing for investigation and gathering of proof, and the administrative wing for registration of complaints and logistics.

Field visits and inspection

Previously, there were no field visits, but now there are regular visits with prior notice given to district and block offices. Karnataka Lokayukta visited all the 176 talukas in 27 districts of Karnataka, including visits to district/taluka hospitals, SC/ST hostels, Anganwadis, remand homes, municipalities, treasury offices and other taluka and district offices. During the visits every day, 100–180 cases of complaints were received and their grievances addressed through public hearings. During inspection, the Lokayukta looks at land and buildings, water and electricity, cleanliness, property encroachment and equipment maintenance. Within human resources, punctuality, vacancies, absenteeism, alcoholism, performance, for example, non-operating surgeons and obstetricians and gynecologists, are examined. Additional qualitative inspection is done on non-clinical services, nursing skills such as bed-making, rational drug use, waste disposal and mortuary and ambulance services. When corrupt practises are noted, the staff member concerned is made to return the bribe amount in full and an oral warning is given. He/she is then monitored by the Administrative Medical Officer, who issues written warnings, if necessary. In case of repetition of offences, the official is charge sheeted and legal proceedings are launched against him/her.

Follow up—inspection notes and compliance

As very little systemic supervision and monitoring exist within the present health care system, empowerment of Administrative

Medical Officers, District Health Officers and other senior staff through capacity building is done. Skill-building in problem-solving, decision-making, facilitation and capacity building and the institution of a citizen's charter are the general measures used for combating corruption.

In one case, an orthopedician at the Kundapura Taluka Hospital had taken bribes for treatment and he was made to return the money. In another notable case, a professor of Community Medicine at a medical college in Bellary took a bribe of Rs 2,500 from 64 students for favours in an examination. The doctor was made to return the bribe amount to the students after subsequent investigation. Corruption is also illustrated by the stocking of unlicensed, imitation drugs throughout Government Medical Stores and in Zilla Panchayats (ZPs) under the Drugs Procurement and Drugs Control Department. The corruption in the procurement of drugs by ZPs is supposedly much more serious in nature. Is decentralised corruption better than centralised corruption?

Corruption in drugs control department

Nearly 50 per cent of pharmacies are without a qualified pharmacist. However, there have been only 14 prosecutions. There was also an incident of HIV positive blood supply from blood bank which did not lead to any prosecution/action due to corruption. The absence of quality standards, including those for falsely licensed or manufactured drugs, is evident, but action is not taken against any of these matters. Many concerns exist regarding sanctioning of illegal loan licenses and product permissions. Due to a violation of Drug Price Control Order (DPCO), the people of Karnataka paid nearly 1 billion in excess and various complaints issued by both the public and by institutions were ignored.

Corruption in procurement of drugs and equipments

Eighteen per cent of the drug procurement budget for Karnataka in 2003 was spent in procuring the drug Nimesulide, a painkiller which is banned in USA and in many countries in Europe. Due to this imbalanced and irrational expenditure, Primary Health Centres (PHCs) were under-stocked or entirely without many essential drugs (such as Paracetamol or Aspirin) while hospitals were stocked with adequate supply of Nimesulide. It is also a well known fact that ministers start their own private drug companies and sell drugs at twice the price to the government itself. A scam involving procurement of IV fluids was executed by bypassing the public-owned company (Hindustan Antibiotics Limited) and buying from a private company instead. Decentralised corruption in ZPs was detected in the procurement of forged, substandard drugs from unlicensed manufacturers at very high prices. Similarly, in the Sigma scam, forged documents of rate contracts fixed by the Directorate General of Supplies and Disposal (DGS&D) were produced.

The Director of Medical Education spent Rs 1.1 million on a dialysis machine worth Rs 500,000, while the Karnataka Institute of Medical Science, Hubli bought the same value machine for Rs 1.2 million. The most notable case was the purchase of equipment for removing cholesterol which was bought for 6 million with consumables worth 75,000 for each cycle. The equipment was bought for the Bowring Hospital and was used only once. Often, the interest shown in procurement does not go even till the installation and procurements are not taken to a logical end. In the case of the Gulbarga ZP X-ray machines were paid for and bought in 1992, but the purchased machines were not installed till 2004, reflecting that purchases are not truly need-based but are simply kickbacks.

Epidemic of corruption in health services

Corruption has roots in many areas—from recruitment to transfers to promotions—and is found at all hierarchical levels, from peons to investigation officers. A typical case of corruption in health services is that of doctors with their own private practise, pharmacies and blood banks and these same doctors usually refer patients to their private nursing homes. All these have led to the doubling of market cost for various health care services, that is, diagnostic or surgical emergency services.

Health sector corruption can be divided in the following ways:

1. Corruption in service delivery by the following: Ayaas/ward boys, contract workers, technicians, administrative staff, nurses, pharmacists, doctors and specialists.
2. Corruption in service delivery for the following services: admission, issuing medical certificates, laboratory investigations, X-ray, scanning, transporting patients and referrals, medical and surgical emergencies, emergency services, elective surgeries, deliveries, blood transfusion and postmortem. Interestingly, corruption insinuates itself into the natural cycle of life and ironically, the lifecycle approach to corruption is what is seen in our country today: it is present at birth, when a relative must pay Rs 200 extra to see the newborn and it is also present at death, when a bribe must be paid for the postmortem.
3. Various forms of corruption by doctors and paramedical staff: Private practise, nursing homes (owned by spouses, relatives and business partners), referrals to private hospitals, owning pharmacies, blood banks, excess of assets over income.
4. Corruption in civil works: Found in construction and repair of PHCs, Community Health Centres (CHCs), Taluka and district hospitals.
5. Corruption in administration: Found in offices at the level of District Health, Directorate and Secretariat for reasons related to recruitment and posting in cities/hometowns, promotion and transfer, leave sanctions, medical reimbursement, monitoring of external private practise, absenteeism, suspension and reinstatement.
6. Corruption in medical education: In sanctioning of new medical, nursing and Indian System of Medicine and Homeopathy (ISM&H) Colleges, in seat increases for nursing colleges, in admissions, in examinations, via bribes for undergraduate and post-graduate examiners, and in recruitment of teaching staff and registration.

Corruption in private sector

In this regard, private hospitals are not very different from the public sector. Many multinational companies have started giving bribes as a means of acquisition of contracts. Commissions are given to doctors for prescription of specific tests/drugs. It is also a standard practice to give 'cuts' for prescription of expensive diagnostic investigations like CT scans and MRIs. In some cases, laboratories run only a few tests and fill in normal values for the rest based on a code with the prescribing doctor, and collect charges for all the tests. Extensive organ trading has occurred earlier in Bangalore and more than 1,000 unrelated kidney transplants bought from the poor people were reported in 1999–2002. Sex selective abortion is also a serious problem in a few districts of Karnataka.

Reforms in health services

After a review of the situation, a few health sector reforms were developed to reduce corruption. Reforms by the Drug Logistic Society led to improvements in obtaining essential drugs that made such drugs available in all PHCs and hospitals. Significant improvements were observed in the number of health staff staying in headquarters through efficient District Health Officers with leadership qualities. Corruption was reduced in equipment purchases due to enhanced vigilance.

More reform for good governance of health services has been initiated in a variety of ways, with a pro-active Lokayukta visiting all the 176 Talukas and institutionalising the reforms. Vigilance cells within the health department have been developed, while e-governance initiatives (such as computerisation and web display of transfers, recruitment, policy-based promotion and purchasing) play a significant role in preventing corruption through transparency and accountability. In all, I visited over 1,200 PHCs and all the Community Health Centres (CHCs), Taluka and District Hospitals in Karnataka and not a single medical officer could tell the budget of his/her institution. Capacity-building in health and hospital management, leadership, decision-making, and problem solving are very important in improving the systems within our health care institutions. In addition, initiatives for staff welfare, improved community participation and monitoring through hospital and health committees, citizen's charter, report card system and public grievance redressal are other measures to counter corruption at the grassroots level.

People's movement for prevention of corruption

The prevention of corruption is however a bottoms-up process, beginning with peoples movement against corruption. It is common knowledge that corrupt people have better networks than people with integrity. There is thus a dire need for networking of people with integrity. In addition, stress on value-based education, awareness of the Right to Information Bill, Transparency Act and Consumer forums needs to be strengthened. Simultaneously, there is a need for electoral reforms so that the gains in the grassroots are not lost at the policy makers level.

Conclusion

As in many other countries, corruption in India is just a passing phase, as evidenced by the changes of the past few years. Today, with the same budget of 800 million for drugs, it is now possible to provide good quality essential drugs to all the primary, secondary and tertiary care health institutions in Karnataka. In a few districts, with good leadership, doctors are staying in headquarters. This is a good sign for our country. Also, various technological packages may produce marginal gains in health care. However, through good governance, a quantum jump of 20–30 per cent improvements in the health outcomes may be attained.

References

Transparency International. 2005. Corruption Perceptions Index 'Transparency International: The Global Collation against Corruption.' Transparency International Secretariat.Germany. Accessed from http://www.un-ngls.org/cso/cso10/corruption.pdf. http://www.transparency.org/policy_research/surveys_indices/cpi, http://www.transparency.org (accessed on 13 September 2007).

Transparency International India. 2005. 'India Corruption Study 2005 to Improve Governance.' Volume 1: Key Highlights. 30 June 2006. Study designed and Conducted by Center for Media Studies. Accessed from http://www.cmsindia.org/cms/events/corruption. pdf; http://www.cmsindia.org/cms/ (accessed on 13 September 2007).

Strategic Leadership and Health Care Delivery 9

Joe Curian

Introduction

Throughout mankind's history, the expectations of what a leader is to achieve have not altered. Even today, with so much industrialisation and technological advancement, the ultimate principles for which a true leader stands have remained unchanged. The aim of this chapter is to focus on leadership in the service sector, particularly within the health care industry.

Uniqueness of health care industry

The health care industry and its unique business model cannot be understood without a description of their background, and the focus of this particular discussion will be against that backdrop. It is important to note, however, that many aspects of leadership are common to all types of industry; leadership is not found solely in health care, since leadership is about leading people. However, health care is part of the service industry and requires special emphasis on certain aspects, and thus understanding the value chain of health care becomes essential (see Figure 9.1).

Like in any other industry, the stages include resources creation, leading to resource mobilisation and then to resource mix and development into products and services on the supply side. The other side is the market (patients). Funding and financing

Figure 9.1 Health care spectrum (value chain)

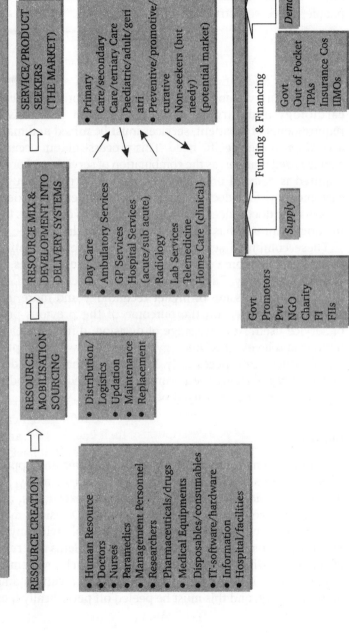

make these two sides interact, transact business and grow. Hospitals are distinct because of the uniqueness of their products, people, processes, structure and technology.

Products

The variety and range of products found in a hospital is incredible, with a vast menu that may include laboratory, radiology, cardiology and surgical services. To meet the individual requirements of a patient, services must be mixed and matched according to the specific need. This process seldom occurs in a standardised manner, as the combination of services and products required is decided only after the patient arrives. Though the customer pays for a doctor's service, the customer is not a decision maker—the doctor decides what is good for his customer. In this, the doctor himself has a stake in the form of doctor's fee.

These combined services often necessitate diagnostic procedures, the outcome of which can require prescriptions, intervention or surgery. Each time, the service occurs as a flexible, graduated progression of higher technology and more intense interventions based on the outcome of the previous product or service used. At every stage of decision, different treatment options and levels of technology are necessary. Consumption of one product often necessarily leads to another. Considerable uncertainty regarding the nature of the subsequent product or service exists for a prolonged period.

People

The hospital environment brings both problems and opportunities, as it deals with knowledge—workers in many fields; doctors, technicians, nursing staff, hospital executives, and financing, marketing and material personnel. Decisions made in a hospital are critical to a degree incomparable with any other business, as hospitals deal routinely with problems that result in life or death. When consistently dealing with such severe matters, human beings unknowingly tend to build up a certain amount of insensitivity, and this must be peeled off periodically if one is to succeed as a health care provider. This is especially important because one invariably meets in addition to the patients, an attendant of the patient who may be a relative or a family member, and compassion is essential. Additionally, the patient must completely trust the provider, as he/she has no means to check whether the full treatment prescribed is truly necessary. The hospital must recognise this and address the psychological aspects of their customer, who is often apprehensive, uncertain and basically uninformed about the value and quality of products or services.

For a care provider, the risks and rewards encountered are disproportionate: a slight error can cause the loss of a patient's life or limb and subsequently result in huge in medico-legal claims. Thus, an expert surgeon or doctor may charge fees that look steep from the patient's perspective.

Doctors

Doctors, unlike other professionals, spend many years acquiring knowledge, developing their skills and garnering expertise before they can claim positions of prominence in their respective fields. A doctor knows that his/her useful time of earning may be limited to 15–20 years, so he/she views every minute and hour as perishable commodities to be converted into high rewards and returns. He/she must make the most of their time, not just to recover the costs incurred but also to make a good return on the significant investment made.

Process

The health care process begins with consulting the doctor about an ailment and can sometimes end in invasive surgery and intensive care in the hospital. The completion of this process may end with the care of the patient in his/her home (see Figure 9.2).

Structure

The organisational structure of a hospital is neither pyramidal, steep, nor flat like a matrix, but is rather like a galaxy where

Figure 9.2   Health care process

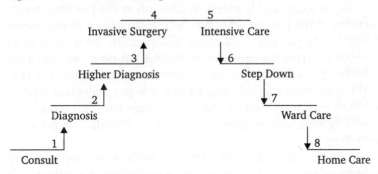

small spheres and clusters comprise a whole system. The locus of control within this galaxy is continually changing. Mission-oriented task forces are created as spherical structures which encompass many methodologies to provide quality service to customers. Each time, unique teams are assembled from a different combination of specialists, doctors, technologists and expert nurses. The component of this structure can be seen in Figure 9.3.

Figure 9.3   Organisational structure of a hospital

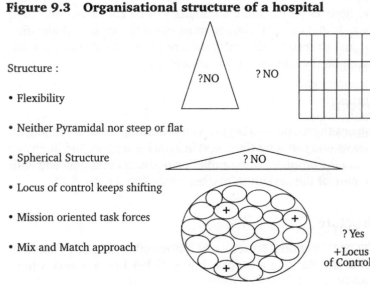

Technology

Nearly 50 per cent of the cost of setting up a new hospital goes into technology. Over 80 per cent of technology has a very short lifespan, as expensive equipment like linear accelerators, gamma knifes, or MRIs may need replacement within six to seven years. However, consumable and disposable goods are estimated to be the largest costs in the health care industry. Globally, the health care industry invests close to four trillion US dollars annually, in all.

Information technology and computerisation has had a great influence on health care. Today, tele-medicine and robotic surgeries are carried out without a patient even seeing a surgeon. New diseases and solutions emerge almost daily, and molecular biology has come to the forefront as an important field. Previously, to diagnose symptoms, doctors would examine the whole body, then a particular organ and then the disease or infection within that organ. Today, however, doctors can examine the particular cell, chromosome, gene and/or sequence of DNA or RNA and use nanotechnology to target drugs.

Quality

Quality is the crux of the hospital industry and this industry has its own economic life that is more or less recession-proof. India, with its population of over 1 billion people and a growing middle class population, is seeing an increase in disposable income and the propensity to spend money on health care. If properly managed and led, hospitals are sure to operate profit-ably, especially since the health care industry is more or less devoid of trend-guided consumption. Instead, there is only a steady stream of customers seeking preventive health care check-ups or diagnostic or curative care depending upon their lifestyle, environment, age and hereditary profile.

Leaders in health care

The qualities needed in a leader may not be different for a leader in the hospital industry as compared to other industries.

However, the intensity of involvement and the commitment to be harnessed from one's team members when dealing with human life is at an entirely different level. When talking about qualities of a good leader, one or more of the following three aspects flash in one's mind:

1. What is he or she?
2. What does he or she do?
3. What has he or she achieved?

What is he?

A Leader is a dreamer

A leader is a dreamer and creative thinker who is constantly conjuring new forms, patterns and colours of systems, processes, products, markets and models of business. He is an artist who uses scientific and methodical practises to implement his dreams. Usually, great leaders experience events twice: first, they perceive the environment in terms of both time and space, and second, they experience the event as plans are implemented.

Leaders predict the occurrence of events ahead of time and therefore look well prepared and brilliant when the actual time comes. In comparison, many of us cannot look ahead in time and are thus not as well equipped to be leaders. The other side of this coin is the spatial dimension: some people look only at their own environment while some others are able to go beyond the boundaries of their little territory. But, great leaders can see not only the whole country but also the world in its entirety, along with the emerging needs and opportunities that accompany each.

Keeps himself well informed

In keeping themselves knowledgeable about political, economic and social issues as well as technological innovation, leaders can perceive future scientific development in other industries and predict the impact of new products on life and environment.

Strategic leadership is all about the ability to understand and nourish the needs of society or a business entity and in response, to create products and services to fill those voids. Every need of the society is viewed as an opportunity and every void as a challenge and invitation. Leaders who understand these voids, seize opportunities and develop innovative ideas that translate into products and services which are embraced by the community, and in this, health care is not an exception. Most leaders have two different facets: creativity as a visionary or thinker and also as a simultaneous achiever who relates to people, who is decisive and appears at the very point where the problem lies. Those born with both these traits can be called brilliant, but a leader born with just one of these traits can learn the other skill. Strategic leadership is the ability to see challenges, destroy existing paradigms and create new paradigms from the component parts for the future.

Important intangibles in strategic success are integrity, a value system that creates a context or ambience of trust, people's motivation, training, creativity, risk profiles and most importantly, across-the-board leadership (see Figure 9.4).

Figure 9.4   Strategic success

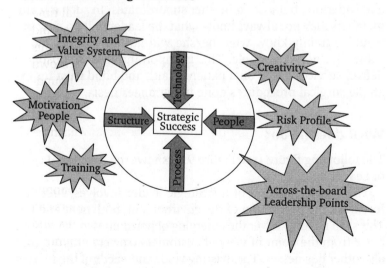

Leaders are radicals

Leaders question current status-quos with their understanding of what lies beyond boundaries. They push not only their own potential beyond the limits set by tradition, but also the other members of their team. In sum, the ability to facilitate new paradigms and mindsets for a team is essential to strategic leadership.

A big heart

Leaders have wisdom consisting of knowledge tempered with experience. They have not only a solid head on their shoulders, but they also always have a big heart and positive attitude. A leader should be able to relate to different strata of people, speak in their language and be able to lead from the front whenever required, to bring out the best in people. He/she must learn to celebrate not just the big accomplishments but also the small victories, and should make an ordinary worker feel like a hero.

Integrity

The single most important personal attribute of a leader is integrity. The value system that a leader possesses is a force not only for instilling confidence and trust among his colleagues and superiors, but also in his/her subordinates. In such a team, members may not always know what the leader will do next but would certainly know what he/she will not do: his/her moral values are non-negotiable. This is important because hospitals deliver services based on a patient's faith and blind trust for example surgical procedures done under anaesthesia.

What does he do?

The following figure (see Figure 9.5) shows the functional cycle of Leadership.

The typical function of a strategic leader involves, first and foremost, the perception of the environment, both near and far. This shall not only cover the emerging opportunities in the market place from the point of view of customers (society at large) but also other businesses. The existing voids and needs of the market would help him to conceive ideas and plans pertaining to new

Figure 9.5   Typical functional cycle of leadership

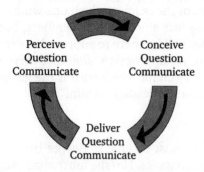

Perceive   Conceive
Question   Question
Communicate   Communicate

Deliver
Question
Communicate

- Perceive-Question-Communicate (PQC)
- Conceive-Question-Communicate (CQC)
- Deliver-Question-Communicate (DQC)

products, services or systems of delivery. It is based on these ideas that products and services should be created, systems iterated and services delivered. Once this is done the market perception on these products/services shall be sought which will result in the said functions assuming a cyclic wherein the same process is repeated.

This can be said to be the perpetual functional cycle of a strategic leader.

Motivation

Selecting the right people for a team and motivating the members selected is a critical issue. A team member's motivation will initially arise from learning the skills needed for a job and the knowledge related to facts. It is thus the duty of a true leader to constantly teach his team—how to win, not only as individuals, but also as a team. For a leader, learning is a constant and continuous activity and through learning, he/she gains the power of knowledge. His or her appetite to learn never ends, as a leader realises that what he or she knows is little compared to the amount of knowledge yet to be acquired. A leader must be well-rounded though he may not be 'a jack of all trades'. For expert advice, he/she should consult the specialists concerned. Human motivation is triggered by individual pride: pride for

one's profession, one's people, one's value system and pride for
the institution or the team in which one works. It is necessary to
build trust not just among team members, but also in the fact
that the leader will be there to support his team, particularly in
times of need. An appropriate simile of these factors is that of
knowledge as a gun for which trust is the gunpowder and pride
is the trigger for motivating a team.

Focus

A leader today must be able to devote time and effort to both
macro and micro issues. He/she must seize every opportunity to
lead by example and demonstrate how to go into detail without
getting involved in the routine operation of an organisation.
Focus must remain not just on broad organisational goals but
also on achieving individual goals, and a leader should endeavour
to unite the two.

Decision-making

Many leaders find that the moment in which decisions must be
made is the loneliest. The plethora of information and abundance
of opinions, discussions and debate can push a leader to a point
that would threaten the weak minded. Yet the instant in which
decisions are made is the moment of truth: today's leaders must
make decisions on the fly, and those made are rarely in black of
white. Decisions reserved for leaders should be those that fall in
the 'grey' area between conflicting choices, and if the decision is
not so, then it is not a decision meant for a leader. The challenge
of such a decision is the eternal truth in a hospital, whether for
the doctors, the executives or the CEO.

Delegate and resolve conflicts

Only through delegation, can a leader find time to dream. He
should be approachable, accessible, and able to get involved if
the situation is such that it cannot be handled by subordinates.
Similarly, a leader must be skilful in conflict resolution, as dis-
sonance can occur not only within the team but also between a
team and the external environment. A true leader must be able

to negotiate, as conflict always exists between a leader and his peers, superiors or other team members. Leaders should have the capacity to separate an issue from an individual and then to be able to integrate issues with individuals. Finally, a bold leader must have the guts to say 'sorry' when the fault is his.

What does he achieve?

The person who has never done a single thing wrong is the person who has not done a single thing. A true leader achieves a level where every team member is responsible for himself. Ultimately, it is the people that count, not plans or strategies. The only caution to be heeded is that teaching and learning must precede the motivation to perform. The mistake of attempting and failing is insignificant compared to the crime of never attempting at all, as is not dreaming of things that never were and asking 'why not?'

Leadership of the future

The leadership of the future can be explained with the following five characteristics:

Style

Leadership styles must change with time. Currently, the traditional feudalistic societies and paternalistic families are breaking down and the knowledge gap between old and young is narrowing. In fact, in many respects, the young are more knowledgeable than the old, and this is true also in business organisations. Thus, leadership of the future will not lie just at the top of the organisational pyramid but throughout. A leader of tomorrow may not necessarily have all the answers, but he/she should have all the right questions, and tolerance to ambiguity will be an essential trait. Technology and people management will be the important issues and the leader should be able to create new processes based on co-operation rather than competition.

Process

Leaders of the future should think of integrating internal processes and systems as per external needs. The pace of business is getting faster, life spans of products are getting shorter and markets are expanding beyond national boundaries. A leader of the future must be prepared to offer both mass production and customer specific services, the choice between which will depend on what model will accrue a larger market share with better margins. In the upcoming e-business era, competition will occur in the same business but between two different models, with new models outpacing old.

Structure

Organisational structures will move from pyramidal to spherical structures, within which the locus of control will continually shift. Mission-oriented task forces and flexible teams will be quickly created and dismantled as soon as their specific tasks are accomplished. Faster web-enabled processes will give leaders shorter times in which to react. A leader will have to rely not only on his or her own creativity, but also on that of his team members, to generate new business using new models.

Change

Innovations in technology and communication—particularly information technology—have made business move at a faster pace. Leaders of the future are those who will grab opportunities for change: true leaders perceive change, conceive change and finally deliver change, leading change with change.

Tips to 'two'

There are two parallel approaches of assuming leadership. The first is that to become a leader, a person should observe the positive and negative attributes of the current leader and then assume those attributes that he/she believes is beneficial. However, a long list of undesirable traits will be left as residue and these should serve as a 'beacon light' for the person to note and avoid. This is an excellent method for incoming leaders to uphold integrity and avoid hypocrisy in their leadership.

The next approach occurs as one assumes the responsibility of leadership in a new organisation or institution. As he/she becomes familiar with the new environment, he/she should prepare a list of 'impossible' tasks to serve as an immediate battlefield to be conquered. After challenging these 'impossibles', the leader will soon realise that their difficulty lies only in changing the mindset of low risk-taking team members. Potentially more than 50 per cent of the 'impossible' tasks would be resolved in the year, and perhaps earlier, depending on the dynamism of the leader. An additional 25 per cent would take a bit longer and in the end, theoretically, over 90 per cent of initially 'impossible' tasks would be able to be resolved. The credit for such achievements must be given to the lower cadres. True leadership converts ordinary performers into heroes.

In the end, it can be said that leaders are the link between the past and the future.

References

Coelho, Paulo. 1998. *The Alchemist*. India: HarperCollins Publishers.

College of Defence Management. 1998. *Leadership*. Hand Book Series. Secunderabad, India: College of Defence Management.

Covey, Stephen R. 1992. *The Seven Habits of Highly Effective People*. London: Simon and Schuster Ltd.

Deming, W. Edwards. 1982. *Out of the Crisis*. Cambridge: Cambridge University Press.

Eckert, R. P. 2001. 'Where Leadership Starts', *Business Today*, 10(23): 84–88.

Fradette, Michael and Steve Michuad. 2000. *The Power of Corporate Kinetics*. United Kingdom: Simon and Schuster Ltd.

Kumar, Pradeep. 2003. 'Leadership Secrets', *Business Today*, 12(11): 142.

Nixon, Bruce. 2001. *Making a Difference*. United Kingdom: Management Books 2000 Ltd.

Wee Chow Hou, Khai Sheang Lee Bambang, Walujo Hidajat. 1996. *Sun Tzu—War and Management*. New York: Addison-Wesley Longman Pvt Ltd.

Wee Chow Hou and Lan Luh Luh. 1998. *The 36 Strategies of the Chinese*. Singapore: Addison-Wesley Longman Singapore Pvt Ltd.

Capacity Development: What, Why and How to Meet Future Challenges in Health Management

10

NANCY GEREIN

Introduction

The term 'capacity development' has been used in development language for the last 50 years. However, recent events have led to a new and intensive discussion of the term's meaning and operation. The concept of capacity development has become more prominent due to the challenges and opportunities raised by a variety of factors: changes in the environment and in populations' concerns and expectations, the information revolution, increasing interest in democratisation and widespread decentralisation of government and economic liberalisation. In facing these new issues, governments, universities, Non-Governmental Organisations (NGOs), families and individuals find that their current lack of capacities have led to a greater need for capacity building programmes. Development donors realise that past efforts in capacity building have not had sustained effects, and, in an effort to improve results, stated their commitment to new forms of development assistance in Paris in March 2005 (OECD 2005). This commitment focuses on building partnerships with national governments, which will ensure that governments take leadership of development efforts and have subsequent ownership of the development process and its results.

Strategic issues and challenges in future health management raise many questions regarding the robustness of the health system's ability to meet these challenges. This chapter explores the major national health issues and their implications for capacity development processes. Capacity development for health must meet the more complex and sometimes less apparent future challenges posed by the changing international context, changes in the environment, the double burden of disease faced by many low-income countries and by our growing understanding of the underlying causes of health status (such as the social determinants of health, including inequities in early childhood development, employment and urbanisation).

Definition of capacity development

A major portion of the concept of Capacity Development (CD) comes from donor perspectives and discourses on development assistance. The United Nations defines CD as a process that 'focuses on enhancing the skills, knowledge and social capabilities available to individuals, institutions and social and political systems'. It also 'supports people's integration into knowledge networks that help to sustain these capabilities' (Whyte 2004: 24). The United Nations Development Programme (UNDP), a major global development agency, places CD at the centre of its mandate. UNDP has defined CD as 'the sustainable creation, utilisation and retention of capacity (to perform functions, solve problems and set and achieve goals), in order to reduce poverty, enhance skills, achieve growth, equalise opportunities and enhance people's lives' (Whyte 2004: 24).

For UNDP, capacity development involves multiple levels: individual, organisational, network, societal, regional and country-wide. Definitions of CD typically specify four interrelated dimensions of capacity development. First, there is a need to ensure productivity through development of individual skills. However, as individuals do not operate in a vacuum, their performance is influenced by the environment in which they work, such that the existence of opportunities for meaningful work, shared professional norms, monitoring and/or incentives will influence performance. Therefore, the second dimension demands development of effective organisations, including public bodies, private businesses, NGOs and community groups. Many tasks require coordination across different organisations (for example, coordination between policy makers and implementing agencies or between training agencies and service organisations). This leads to the third dimension, which emphasises strengthening of the inter-relationships or networks between organisations. Last, capacity development focuses on the need for formulation of a systems-oriented approach that creates an environment able to address the cross-sectoral issues that affect society.

History of the concept of capacity development

A historical review of the conceptualisation of CD reveals numerous different 'waves' in the idea's evolution, ranging from institution building to framing of knowledge networks. In 1960s, institution building was the major focus, with emphasis in 1960s–1970s moving toward institutional strengthening focussed on the public sector, individuals and training. During this time models from wealthy countries were transposed to low-income countries. During the 1970s, more weight was given to improving delivery systems, such that public programmes could better reach neglected groups in society. Attention was given to human resource development, targeting especially the health, education and population sectors, during the 1970s–1980s (Whyte 2004). Then, in the 1990s, 'new institutionalism' came into prominence, focusing on structural adjustment and policy change. At this stage, the need was felt to include NGOs and the private sector in capacity building networks. In the most recent conceptual stage, more attention is given to the external, global environment and national economic behaviour, especially the strengthening of national economic and legal institutions that foster the development of private enterprise.

Most recently, with the creation of the Millennium Development Goals, the focus on the role of government has been reinforced,

and the need to make governments more effective is now para-
mount. To advance CD, local ownership, appropriate technical
assistance and participatory approaches were reassessed. More
emphasis is placed on careful needs assessment and analysis,
on systems approaches, Information Communication Technology
(ICT), knowledge networks and on ongoing learning and adap-
tation. Results-based management, sustainability, better donor
coordination and long-term donor investment have also been
recognised as areas needing concentration, in order to realise
the potential of CD.

Shifts in capacity development strategies

Initially, CD focused on the professional skills of individuals; however, this later shifted to organisational and then institutional
competence. Institutional competence refers to the formal rules
of organisational behaviour, while organisational competence
refers to informal norms of behaviour and codes of conduct
followed by people. For differentiating, it can be said that institutions are 'the rules' while organisations are the 'players' of the
game. Prominence was first given to the development of technical
and analytical tools, but has now shifted to policy relevance and
problem-solving of the real issues of organisations and systems.
CD was initially concerned with the production of professionals
but did not consider the productivity of those professionals produced. Another change required was to review the interaction
of individual organisation with multiple organisations. It was
realised that CD cannot be confined to the government sector
alone, since the quality of policy outputs is enhanced through
interaction between governments and the private sector, civil
society, NGOs, universities, quasi-government organisations and
professional organisations.

The focus on different levels of organisational systems is
best illustrated by taking examples from a large development
programme in India. Based on the 1994 Cairo meeting on population and development, the government implemented a new
policy framework for its family welfare sector. During implementation of the new framework, the lack of skills, time, money

and authority were identified as causes for the weakness of the government programmes. The proposed solutions were training and additional development resources (that is, addition of staff, vehicles, sufficient budget, building research institutions and training schools). However, it was eventually realised that professionals (doctors, managers or other staff) were unable to perform effectively, even after the necessary training and facilities were provided, because more deep-rooted problems, the dysfunctional administrative and organisational arrangements remained, systematically undermining an individual's attempts to carry out quality work (Potter and Brough 2004).

In order to overcome these problems, a systematic approach was adopted for CD. Figure 10.1 shows the capacities required for comprehensive system change, illustrating both top-down

Figure 10.1 The required capacities

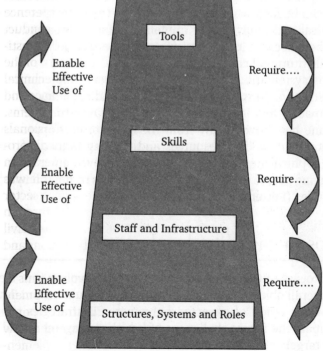

Source: Potter and Brough 2004.

and bottom-up approaches. Using the top-down approach, it can be seen that the use of tools requires skills, skills in turn require capable staff with adequate infrastructure, which in turn requires supportive structures, systems and roles. Viewed from the bottom-up, it is observed that structures, systems and roles enable the effective use of staff and infrastructure, which then enables the effective use of staff skills and available tools.

The basic framework of required capacities (of individuals to systems) influenced the development of a hierarchy of organisational capacity needs (see Figure 10.2). This hierarchy indicates that the effectiveness or performance of one capacity depends upon another. Under this approach, nine components of capacity were identified, starting with performance and personal capacities and moving to workload, supervisory, facility and support service capacities. At the bottom, it is seen that all these elements depend on systems, structural and role capacities. The capacities at the top are technical and development at this level can be fast, whereas at the bottom, the capacities are less technical and imply slower implementation of broad changes. It is these socio-cultural capacities which are closely associated with institutional capacities.

This systematic approach to CD has been implemented in 50 districts of 24 states and territories in India, aiming to develop capacity for decentralised planning. Over time, the programme has moved away from the older project approach to development (adding resources and training individuals) to a more sophisticated approach, which has proved effective in encouraging people to prioritise system changes rather than project initiatives (Potter and Brough 2004).

Steps in capacity development

The process of CD for health management involves four steps. The overall objective is to assess the current situation and develop a clear vision of expected outcomes. CD strategies should anticipate the future challenges of health management and set clear targets for achievement.

Figure 10.2 Organisational capacities

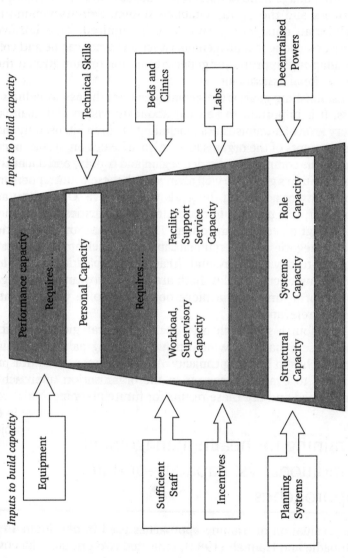

Source: Potter and Brough 2004.

The first step involves determining the current capacities for health management, at the levels of the individual, organisation, network and the overall enabling system. Self-assessment, as well as an outsider's perspective, is required, especially for decision making in management issues. Evidence can be gathered by adapting appropriate generic tools for organisational and institutional assessment.

Establishing goals is the second step after the assessment process. It is important to be clear about the vision and goals for every level of administration, including the individuals, units and departments of the organisation. Also, a health organisation is a part of the community, district, region and country and if a health organisation's goals are well aligned with these counterparts, the possibility of achieving the goals will increase. Once the goals are clear, it is possible to determine the capacities that need to be strengthened—the third step. These can be thought of in two main categories: (*i*) operational capacities which are used to carry out day-to-day activities; and (*ii*) adaptive capacities in response to shifting circumstances. Both are required by an organisation to perform functions, achieve objectives, solve problems and remain relevant.

The fourth step is then to decide the strategies for achieving these capacities, which include training as well as other approaches to building capacity. After implementation, it is important to evaluate changes in the organisation, planned or unplanned and use these results for future planning.

Training for health management: Traditional vs. capacity-oriented approaches

An evaluation of training approaches used in development by Honadle and Hannah (1982), indicated two primary objectives of training—to improve the performance of an organisation and to enhance its ability to function within a changing environment. However, they noted that these objectives are not frequently met because of inadequate approaches: rather than dealing with real organisational problems faced by specific groups and building on skills the trainees already have, standardised training is given to groups of unrelated trainees in a facility using hypothetical examples. Training is offered as a discrete event conducted during one or two days (or even weeks) away from the desk; the learning is promptly forgotten in the rush of e-mails and memos that must be dealt with upon returning to work.

Rather than transferring knowledge to individuals, a more productive method is to take an action-based approach, enhancing capacity to meet an organisation's specific needs. In order to bring about the required organisational change, it is necessary to be clear about the contribution of trained individuals to the organisation. A training plan should include the often forgotten people who carry out support functions, such as administrative and financial procedures, office management (filing, storage, communications) and equipment maintenance (de Savigny et al. 2004). Training should be arranged under convenient conditions. It should be specific, short appropriate and interdisciplinary.

Training should be given to a group or to several crucial personnel, such that an individual is not expected to single-handedly change the organisation. Numerous evaluations of research development programmes have shown that scientific training of individuals is insufficient to achieve sustainable change. Training efforts are undermined by several characteristics of the environment of a research organisation—lack of academic liberty, incentives, research funds, opportunities for scholarly networking and implementation of research projects—which are guided by foreigners' interests rather than by their country's own research priorities. Ongoing professional development and an enabling environment are key to building and maintaining research capacity (Andruchow et al. 2005). These principles are also relevant to non-research organisations.

Last, given the nature of development challenges and potential contributors, it is clear that training and capacity development should involve not only the government and large organisations, but also small businesses and civil society organisations.

Non-training approaches to CD

Non-training approaches include the use of advisers, consultants or resource persons, adopting adult learning formats in workshops and holding meetings, conferences and study tours to educate groups of people. Establishing networks of multidisciplinary institutions—regional, national and international; involving universities, businesses and civil society—which can potentially become centres of excellence, is becoming more common. The provision of information through such networks and through the spread of ICT is critical to CD. At the organisational level, management support for learning, reflection and use of new ideas via coaching and mentoring is necessary. Another innovation is giving sabbaticals, traditionally only conducted in the universities, but which are now considered helpful for other organisations too.

Future challenges in health management

A future challenge for capacity development in health management will be the need for policy makers to take into consideration the enormous growth in knowledge about causes of ill-health and the means of improving it. The new perspectives are frequently complex and traditionally not within the health care sector, for example, the social determinants of health: what is the role of the Ministry in dealing with poverty, poor housing and dangerous jobs? The increasing complexity in health conditions is matched by the growing intricacy in the organisation, financing and management of health care systems (Frenck 2006). The growth of and changes in information and technology will create many new ethical issues in health, both at the individual (clinical care) and population levels (for example, setting priorities and dealing with gender and equity issues). All these changes signify that organisations will need to obtain and manage a greater diversity of skills and disciplines, either within the organisation or through inter-organisational relationships.

Another challenge faced by health systems is globalisation. The management of globalisation requires an understanding of its implications, which are traditionally in the area of epidemiology and the control of diseases, but now go well beyond to include issues raised by free trade and the greater mobility of professionals and multinationals across borders. The implications of these trends for population health will require the Ministry of Health (MoH) to collaborate with different ministries, such as Trade, Labour and Finance and to learn a new language which advocates effectively for the protection and promotion of health, in a context of free trade and globalisation (Vellinga 2002).

Human Resources (HR) are gaining their rightful prominence in the development of health systems. Health systems must develop more professional human resource management systems. All too often, HR management is isolated and under-professionalised, with the result that, planning and forecasting of HR needs, and good management of existing HR, does not occur. Given the competition for HR from richer countries and from better-paid employment sectors within countries, it will be critically important to find ways to attract young people to health services and to retain them (Joint Learning Initiative 2004).

Another change implied is that MoHs will have to focus not only on their own organisation and on the role of other government departments, but also on making the best use of and indeed enlarging, the capacities of the wider health system. This system will include other government sectors, the private sector, and a large number of civil society organisation, communities, individuals and families. Building of the community's capacities for health especially requires a great deal of participation and leadership, as well as proper organisational structures, problem assessment skills. And effective resources mobilisation (Gibbon et al. 2002). MoHs will need to improve the health system's resources by building partnerships need to be appropriately managed, requiring organisational commitment and incentives for staff to take on these roles.

Both the adaptive and operational capacities that will be needed are considerable. Given that many of these challenges are not traditionally the purview of the MoH, and are not within the main current policy areas or managerial spans of control, the challenges to health managers are compelling even now, and therefore will be even more so in the future.

Analysis of the CD approaches and goals indicates that information and evidence from evaluation is another challenging issue. Rigorous research and evaluation is important to persuade politicians to continue with effective health innovations and to inform programme decision-making (Frenk 2006). It is also key to understanding what capacities can be developed through the most effective approaches. For example, does training for executive board members result in specific skill improvements that result in higher quality programmes and services? Since capacity building is not a simple 'cause and effect' process, there is still a need to generate innovative approaches that will fulfil the needs of CD under many circumstances, and to assess the outcomes of these carefully, to build up a body of evidence on 'what works', at the level of the individual, department, organisation and system.

The area of focus of MoH activities may change with time, but the main objective remains the improvement (development) of the population's health. Because of the growing disciplinary skill-set needed by MoHs to meet the future challenges described above, a change from clinician managers to professional managers is inevitable. These managers will need to find ways that enable all individuals in the organisation to function at their highest potential capacity—to create, in effect, a 'capacity releasing' organisation.

References

Andruchow, J. E., C. L. Soskolne, F. Racioppi and R. Bertollini. 2005. 'Capacity building for epidemiologic research: a case study in the newly independent state of Azerbaijan', *Annals of Epidemiology*, 15(3): 228–231.

de Savigny, D., H. Kasale, C. Mbuya and G. Reid. 2004. *Fixing Health Systems*. Ottawa: International Development Research Centre.

Frenk, J. 2006. 'Bridging the divide: global lessons from evidence-based health policy in Mexico', *The Lancet*, 368(9539): 954–961.

Gibbon M., R. Labonte, G. Laverack. 2002. 'Evaluating community capacity', *Health and Social Care in the Community*, 10(6): 485–491.

Honadle, G. H. and J. P. Hannah. 1982. 'Management performance for rural development: packaged training or capacity building', *Public Administration and Development*, 2(4): 295–307.

Joint Learning Initiative Strategy Report. 2004. *Human Resources for Health: Overcoming the Crisis*. Cambridge, Massachusetts: Harvard University Press.

OECD/DAC. 2005. 'Paris Declaration on Aid Effectiveness: Ownership, Harmonisation, Alignment, Results and Mutual Accountability.' Organisation for Economic Cooperation and Development, Development Assistance Committee. Accessed from http://www.oecd.org/dataoecd/11/41/34428351.pdf (accessed on 18 September 2007).

Potter, C. and R. Brough. 2004. 'Systematic Capacity Building: A Hierarchy of Needs', *Health Policy and Planning*, 19(5): 336–345.

Vellinga, J. 2002. 'An Approach to Trade and Health at Health Canada', in C. Vieira and N. Drager (eds), *Trade in Health Services: Global, Regional, and Country Perspectives*, pp. 193–96. Washington: Pan American Health Organization.

Whyte, A. 2004. 'Landscape Analysis of Donor Trends in International Development', A Rockefeller Foundation Series, Issue No. 2, New York. (Available online at http://www.rockfound.org/Documents/707/hicb_whyte_donortrends.pdf).

Capacity Development Model in Enhancing Health Care (Eye Care) Services—The Aravind Eye Care Model

11

KEERTI BHUSAN PRADHAN

Introduction

Every 5 seconds, one person in this world goes blind. Globally, 45 million people are blind, 135 million are visually impaired and 90 per cent of these people live in the developing world. However, out of this, 80 per cent of blindness can be avoided. In India, with its population of 1 billion, 112 million people are blind, and each year, 6 million new people develop blindness from cataract, though it is an avoidable disease. Eye care is cost effective—as per the World Bank statistics, the yearly cost of blindness in India is around US dollars 30 million. In the year 2004, 4,500,000 surgeries were performed in India, but a gap exists between the need and availability of services.

In a developing country where demands compete for limited resources, the government alone cannot meet all of the poor's health needs. In response to the urgent need for care, Dr G. Venktaswamy started an 11-bed eye clinic to create an alternate, sustainable eye care system as a supplement to government efforts. This hospital is named after Sri Aurobindo Ghosh, whose teachings form the basis of the hospital's work. The values incorporated into the hospital's practice are equity, compassion, transparency and integrity.

Aravind Eye Hospital (AEH) is the world's largest eye hospital, with more than 4,000 beds and 250,000 eye surgeries performed each year. The elements of the Aravind eye care system are il-lustrated in Figure 11.1, and the mission of the Aravind Eye Care System is to eliminate needless blindness through the provision of compassionate and high quality care to all. The first clinic was started in 1978 in Madurai and there are now several branches of Aravind Eye Hospitals. The Theni branch (1984) is a small clinic that serves as a model for all developing countries and for people who evaluate and study capacity building programmes. Other centers are in Tirunelveli (1988), Coimbatore (1997) and Pondicherry (2003). All the Aravind Eye Hospitals have been instituted and have sustained growth without the aid of external or international grants—development funds are solely provided by internal income, and additionally, 65 per cent of services are provided free of cost.

Figure 11.1   Aravind eye care system–elements

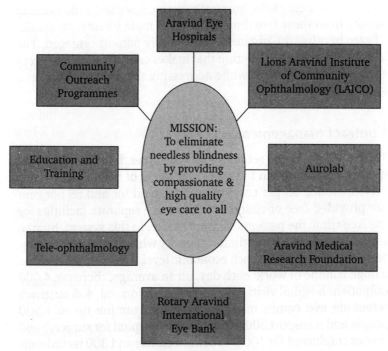

Sources: The Fortune at the Bottom of the Pyramid.
C.K. Prahalad, *The Fortune at the Bottom of the Pyramid*, p. 266. Wharton School Publishing.

Aravind eye hospital—service model and operational model

The Aravind Eye Care System, which today is the largest eye care facility in the world, demonstrates that it is possible to effectively combine low cost, high quality, world scale and sustainability. This hospital is a good model of a non-profit organisation from which others can learn, but one must view the hospital from two dimensions to get a complete perspective. The first dimension is as a 'unique business model'—most organisations are market driven, whereas this hospital utilises a market driving approach which focuses on latent needs. As a result, the hospital has developed its own market and made its services affordable and accessible to all. The second dimension is the spiritual or greater purpose within which the 'business model' operates, and the effectiveness of the hospital's work comes from the synergy arising from these two dimensions. The main focus is on quality of care because the organisation is purely patient centered. The system has a pricing structure that makes care affordable to every segment of the society, while addressing the aspect of financial sustainability.

Contract management

The hospital provide service at specified fees, but the values and quality of care remain the same regardless of the charge. In this service model, 35 per cent services are paid for and 65 per cent are provided free-of-charge and there are separate facilities for the free clinic the patients may opt to use. In this system, human resources are used for optimum capacity while the facilities themselves are designed for each economic level. The hospital handles a huge volume of work: each day, on an average, there are 4,000 outpatient hospital visits, 750 surgeries performed, 4–5 outreach screening eye camps organised (which examine up to 1,500 people and transport 300 patients to the hospital for surgery) and classes conducted for 100 Residents/Fellows and 300 technicians and administrators.

Community outreach

Community outreach is a core philosophy and community partners implement the majority of programmes. In a state with a population of 65 million, 15,000 community partners organise 20–25 camps per week that register patients, conduct free surgeries and provide food, transportation and other services. The hospital places strong emphasis on community participation, which indirectly results in much lower human resource cost to the organisation. The hospital has achieved its success because it does not directly treat the community but instead uses the help of various community partners to provide care. Additionally, referral services are also provided by the hospital.

The hospital has also started conducting diabetic retinopathy camps in partnership with communities and nephrologists since diabetic patients need regular check ups and these camps can foster awareness. Refraction services that provide comprehensive eye screening and refractive error service at the same location have recently been implemented. Prescriptions are provided free of cost in a highly efficient manner: once the patient receives the prescription from the doctor, 85 per cent of spectacles are directly delivered within half an hour. In a partnership with schools, the institution provides eye care services for children in a novel way—schoolteachers are trained on how to conduct preliminary screenings, and the teachers then refer students to the ophthalmologist. Later, diagnostic and refraction services are provided to the children with additional follow-up occurring. As a globally recognised institution committed to excellence, the AEHs constantly search for innovative approaches to enhance their intellectual growth and not-for-profit business model. Top universities and business schools have sought the expertise of AEH and used its unique non-profit management model as an educational example for their students.

Productivity

Forty per cent of all cataract surgeries in Tamil Nadu are performed in AEHs. A single surgeon in this hospital performs more than 2,000 cataract surgeries in a year, which is five times the number performed by the average Indian ophthalmologist. Altogether, in one year the hospitals perform 150,000 cataract operations, which is more than the total measured by the entire National Health Survey (NHS) (Mark Tully, BBC 2002). During 2005, surgeries were conducted and the system screened more than 1.63 million people on an outpatient basis. It conducted more than 1,150 eye camps in southern India, and since 1976, the number of surgeries has substantially increased—as of 2005, an estimated surgeries have been performed in AEHs.

At the same time, the hospital is extending the coverage of quality eye care to remote villages in South India. This is being done through village internet kiosks—Information Technology (IT) is utilised to increase accessibility and telemedicine is used to provide the best care for patients. Realising the cost of imported consumables goods, AEH began manufacturing its own eye care products and by doing so, the prices for intraocular lenses have came down from US dollars 100 to US dollars 2, thus making cataract surgery affordable. Additionally, the hospital is currently exporting the product to the 120 countries all over the world.

Lions Aravind Institute of Community Ophthalmology (LAICO)

There was a need to institute capacity building, as the hospital works to act as a model system. The problems initially experienced in treating blindness was lack of appropriately trained manpower, proper systems and procedures and community buy-in. Therefore, replicating the lessons learnt at the hospital could be used to address some of the above issues on a bigger scale. Realising the success of its system, AEH decided to share its experience with other eye care programmes such that the common mission of 'eliminating needless blindness' and the goal of 'preventing and controlling global blindness through teaching, training, consultancy, research, publication and advocacy' could be reached throughout the world. This was initially executed informally, with the demand from other eye care organisations determining the extent of study of the AEH system. Due to increasing demand, AEH officially established LAICO with the support of Lions Club International. As a result, Aravind Eye Care System now offers a wide range of training designed to enhance the management capacity of other eye hospitals and eye care programmes. LAICO is also helping to build capacity into eye care services in 30 other African, Asian and Latin American countries through training, consultancy, networking and observational visits. To date, the institute has trained more than 1,100 cataract trainees from different parts of the world.

This organisation is a growing resource of eye care service management for supporting eye care services through government, private and charity sectors. This model must also be analysed to determine its applicability in other service sectors to improve the utilisation, quality, sustainability and management of services through evidence-based management practises. LAICO offers courses that have university affiliation with regular training programmes. The courses are specialised in eye care management. Some of the courses include 'Management Priorities in Eye Care Delivery', 'Eye Care Programme Managers', 'Management of Eye Hospitals', 'Clinical & Supervisory Skill Development for Ophthalmic Paramedics', 'Optical Dispensing', 'Instruments Maintenance for Technicians' and 'Community Outreach'. Additionally, upon realising the need for eye care management, LAICO introduced a one-year fellowship course in eye care management.

Capacity building through consultancy

The Manpower and Management Development Programme was started to enhance the capacity of eye hospitals. It focussed on solving funding issues in eye care delivery by building long-term financial viability through patient revenues. The objectives of the manpower and management development programme are as follows:

1. to help hospital leadership articulate a well-defined vision and goal for their hospital,

2. to assist in developing an efficient and cost effective system that will provide high volume, good quality cataract surgery at affordable cost,
3. to make hospitals financially sustainable through patient revenues, and
4. to provide the necessary clinical and management training to hospital personnel.

By promoting the adoption of relevant technologies and skill perspectives through international visits and exchanges, this programme seeks to constantly improve the quality of services provided. Continuous improvements are made based on patient and employee feedback. From time to time, the hospital conducts trainings for residents from leading US institutions. Apart from this, it performs teaching and training programmes for technicians, ophthalmologists and administrators. The hospital has 40 structured and well-designed training programmes per year and has trained 1,120 doctors from 30 countries, including 928 from India. Classes for 100 Residents/Fellows and 300 technicians and administrators are run simultaneously, making AEH the largest provider of eye care services and trainer of ophthalmic personnel in the world. While promoting internal capacity building programmes, volunteers from different countries help transfer external skills. Additionally, conferences, in-house training programmes, meetings and presentations are organised for sharing information and knowledge, with regular updates distributed.

Fees are structured such that poor people pay nothing and financially able patients pay just $1 for a visit to the outpatient clinic. Depending on the type of surgery and facility necessary, 40 per cent of patients pay between $50–150, which is comparably favourable to the $3,000–3,500 charged for a similar operation in the US. This system has proved to be profitable, as the net surplus is about 45 per cent of the revenue and this is accomplished without compromising quality. A comparison of quality of care in AEH to that of quality of eye care in UK (where the Royal Ophthalmic Society published the results of a survey of over 18,000 surgeries) shows that AEH overcame every medical parameter of complications during the operation and in post-operation, as based on evidence from 22,000 surgeries. Ophthalmologists working at AEH are almost 10 times as efficient as the national average.

The initial step for capacity building is to select a hospital, and to then collect data about the specified hospital by performing a needs assessment. Once this is accomplished, a field visit to the hospital must be made to develop a strategic action plan (SAP), with support throughout the procedure from heads of departments such as nursing and medicine. Based on information from the needs assessment and SAP, the institute will train hospital staff, over the course of a week, on implementing the programmes in the hospital. Follow-up is made and assistance is provided in case the hospital faces problems. Throughout the whole process, monitoring and feedback mechanisms operate to measure the progress of the consultancy provided.

Consultancy for capacity building

The institute has extended its collaboration with various international agencies such as Lions Club International Foundation; Sight Savers International, UK; CBM International, Germany; Seva Foundation, USA; International Eye Foundation, USA; WHO; ORBIS International, USA; and Dark & Light, Netherlands, for providing funding to training programmes. Recently, direct requests have been received from individual eye hospitals soliciting training programmes.

A government hospital of Malawi (Malawi Eye Care Project) is an example where substantial growth in surgeries was demonstrated. The main objectives of this project were to:

1. develop the hospital's capacity to make it a high quality centre for eye care services in Malawi,
2. train human resources and personnel in skill development regarding both clinical and management functions,
3. support the design and development of systems and processes for better functioning of the hospital, and
4. ensure financial sustainability through improved strategies for both paying and free services.

After intervention and a successful capacity building programme, a considerable increase in the OPD, camps and surgeries
performed per year was observed. Before AEH's intervention, the
Malawi Eye Care Project conducted 449 IOL surgeries in 1998,
while now as many as 500 surgeries can be performed in five
weeks. Currently, 3,000 surgeries are performed per year by the
same team of doctors. Increasing the number of surgeries could
become possible after establishing the systems for outreach,
clinical and administrative protocols and improving management strategies.

The impact of capacity building training was observed within
two years of the workshop, when the total number of cataract
surgeries performed in 40 hospitals in India increased from
52,506 to 91,445 per year. Additionally, the number of surgeries
per ophthalmologist increased from 448 to 848, with surgeries
per bed increasing from 33 to 49 during the specified period.
Similarly, cost recovery, which was only 70 per cent, has gone
up to 90 per cent two years after the workshop (see Table 11.1).
All these processes indicate that structured capacity building is
a sustainable, cost-effective strategy that can increase the level
of eye care services over a short time period. This process becomes very effective when the required enabling conditions
(leadership, attitude and staff) are in place.

**Table 11.1   Impact of capacity building process (Resource
utilisation)**

Total cataract surgeries	1 yr before workshop	2 yr after workshop	Increase %
Total Cataract Surgeries	52,506	91,445	74%
Cost Recovery	71%	90%	27%
Surgeries per Ophthalmologist	448	848	89%
Surgeries per Bed	33	49	48%

Source: Case Study by Professor S. Manikutty and Professor Neharika Vohra,
IIM Ahmedabad.

Not all hospitals that have been trained are performing well;
yet the improved hospitals reveal that some essential factors have
contributed to their phenomenal success. These factors involve
committed leadership, dedicated and trained staff, quality of

medical/surgical care, employment of a full-time ophthalmologist, organised outreach programmes, focussed screening camps, community involvement, effective counselling, housing of all services under one roof, service differentiation, cost control, professional administration, the number of OPDs and surgeries per day, streamlined work flow, need-based investments and continuous training and development. On the other hand, some of the weakness that hampered a hospital's performance after the workshop were: frequent change in leadership; employment of a part-time ophthalmologist; frequent turnover of ophthalmologists; inferior quality of medical/surgical care; absence of outreach programmes, counselling, service differentiation and emotional investment; limited surgery days and OPD timings; and lack of professional administration.

Capacity building development was done at an organisational level with a focus on cataract & refractive error services, paediatric ophthalmologic services (partners of International Nongovernmental Organisations [INGOs]), diabetic retinopathy services (partners of INGOs), instruments maintenance training (Nigeria, Vietnam, Kenya), management training, Kilimanjaro Centre for Community Ophthalmology (KCCO–Tanzania) and contract management. Residency training programmes for improving teaching at hospitals had generally focussed on private hospitals, but now the focus has shifted to incorporate government hospitals as a result of so much organisational support for the training programmes (that is, Project Management). In addition to this, the institute has developed a software tool named 'Integrated Hospital Management Systems' for managing patient care-related activities, managing selected administrative areas in a hospital and for generating information regarding day-to-day management, decision-making and clinical quality assurance. However, in spite of all these interventions, 37,000,000 people are still become blind (time frame).

The experience of AEH shows that capacity building can holistically reach the unserved sectors of society. It is appropriate to note that 'health initiatives in developing countries often fail not because of a lack of scientific knowledge but because of a lack of managerial competence' (Dr Mike Malison, CDC-Atlanta, SMDP).

Conclusion

Many lessons were learned from the activities of LAICO-Aravind Eye Hospitals. These systems were designed to improve collaboration between developing countries and build their internal capacities such that their reliance on technical assistance from developed countries could be lessened. The most common approaches utilised between these developing partners are networking, study tours, visits, technical assistance, training, meetings and conferences. LAICO suggests that these approaches (or a combination thereof) should be initiated and driven by the needs of the country and region receiving the assistance, instead of by requirements from the donor agency. Regardless of the developing partner's approaches, LAICO has revealed that it is important to have clearly identified objectives, appropriate participants, long-term relationships between partners, and, where necessary, some level of continued donor funding. Collaboration between developing partners is a long-term investment in programmatic sustainability that requires one to establish and maintain long-term relationships. It involves both exchange between developed partners and capacity development, when needed. Such collaborations have the potential to build local or regional infrastructure and skills that contribute to technical, programmatic and institutional sustainability. Findings from this review should be useful to the members of international donor agencies with its provision of recommendations for incorporating S-to-S collaboration in all funded development projects through identification of key resource organisations among the developing countries.

References

Annual Report. 2006. *Aravind Eye Care System*.

Kasturirangan, V. *In Service for Sight*. Harvard Business School Case Study, The Aravind Eye Hospital, Madurai, India.

Man's World. 2002. 'The Spirit of the Millennium Man', *Man's World*, October.

Shah, Janat and L. S. Murthy. 2004. 'Compassionate, High Quality Health Care at Low Cost: The Aravind Model', *IIMB Management Review*, 16(3).

Managing AIDS Control Programme in India

12

RAJEEV SADANANDAN

Introduction

India is set to implement the third phase of the National AIDS Control Programme from the next financial year. The current scenario is very different from what existed when the first phase was started in 1992, when there was 'very little mobilisation against HIV/AIDS and much denial of its impact' (NACO 1999a). At least one authority has claimed that India has the largest number of persons infected with HIV, even though prevalence levels are lower than in many other countries (UNAIDS 2006). The programme has demonstrated success in southern and western parts of the country while the situation in North India remains grim (Kumar et al. 2006). The level of funding has been on the increase. While the civil society, including persons infected and affected by the disease, continues to clamour for greater involvement in the programme, the medical systems are increasingly engaged and demand a greater share of resources. It is now recognised that unless all sectors are involved, a reduction in the epidemic may not be achieved or sustained. Given the size of the programme, it will be necessary to decentralise management to districts and lower levels. Such conditions make the management of the new phase of the AIDS Control Programme a bigger challenge than before. Whether the programme will achieve its objectives or not will depend on the degree to which appropriate attitudes and systems are developed to meet this challenge.

Global response to HIV

Management systems for AIDS prevention and control differ from other public health programmes. This is partly explained by the history of AIDS, which is a fairly recent epidemic. HIV was first noticed among the gay population of USA. At the time of impact the medical community was not equipped to deal with the new virus. The only response came from the gay community. They had already mobilised themselves to fight discrimination and win political and social acceptance. They now turned to their cadres to encourage safe behaviour, fight discrimination and mitigate the impact of the disease. This brought in new players and new systems, setting up models of programme management which have become the standard in the rest of the world. It also gave the civil society an undeniable role in the response to AIDS. Globalisation ensured that systems developed in the developed countries were carried to other parts of the world to become part of the response from the beginning.

After initial bewilderment, the medical community responded with energy. HIV has seen some of the fastest strides in medical and pharmacological research. Many committed members of the medical community recognised the need to manage opportunistic infections that followed infection by HIV. Treatment of Sexually Transmitted Infections (STIs) was also perceived as an effective prevention strategy. By 1990s, the first drug for anti-retroviral treatment had been approved. Since then AIDS has seen an increasing role for the biomedical sector. When generic drugs were made available for anti-retroviral therapy, the poor of the world had increased access to medical care. But this increased the management load on National AIDS Control bodies who were finding it difficult to cope with the demand for increased prevention services. Therefore, unlike other disease control programmes, the HIV/AIDS strategies have both non-health and health components and their integration has been and will continue to be a major challenge.

Response in India

In India too the first response in prevention came from the civil society, inspired and supported by global civil society networks. Non-Govermental Organisations (NGOs) received technical support and funding from international organisations. Given the moral and social baggage attached to the disease, established public health activists kept away from the programme. The resulting vacuum was filled by young and non-traditional activists. This led to an openness to ideas which may not otherwise have been received enthusiastically, thereby leading to unconventional strategies in the AIDS control programmes. Their openness was to influence the government strategies as many of the activists were involved in designing the government-led national programmes.

Some factors that have shaped AIDS Programme in India

Geographical

It may have been fortuitous that the states where the virus was first noticed also had good governance and health systems. Consequently they were able to implement most of the prevention components successfully. Being initial adopters and since they could absorb external support, these states also had access to national and international technical assistance. Combining these advantages, they were able to develop AIDS control models appropriate to their situations and needs. A model, abstracted from these successes, was subsequently adopted as the national one and applied to all the states in India (NACO 1999b: 9). But given the differences between the health systems of the different states, those with weak governance systems have not been able to replicate the performance of the early adopters.

Unfortunately some of the underperforming states have a history of being the largest reservoir of all major communicable diseases in the country. These were the last pockets to fall in small pox eradication. The Global Polio Eradication programme is yet to succeed here. Kala Azar and Leprosy remain endemic. A significant percentage of population continues to suffer from Malaria and TB. These states have populations larger than most countries in the world and extremely poor health and other social indicators. The AIDS programme presupposes collaboration with active civil society organisations. Past history of collaboration between such organisations and governments has not been very happy. The deficit of goodwill and trust is not a good platform for dealing with the challenges of AIDS control programme. These states appear not to be mounting an effective response to the epidemic. The impact could be catastrophic on their poor populations and the total number of infected persons in the country.

The geographical proximity of the north eastern states to South East Asia not only linked them as part of the drug route but also in the injection mediated epidemic that characterised South Asia. The epidemic in the north east therefore differed from the rest of the country, where AIDS is spread mainly through the sexual route. Since the efficiency of transmission is many times higher through the injecting route, north eastern states of Manipur and Nagaland and later Mizoram saw a runaway epidemic. The response in these states is hampered by a scattered health care system, civil unrest and distance from the centre of decision-making in Delhi. One of the strategies that will be attempted is to decentralise decision-making to a unit of NACO set up in the north east.

Sociological

HIV is driven by many factors, most of which are stigmatised and some of which are illegal. The Indian middle class, which constitutes the most significant proportion of the governing class in the country, is uncomfortable with issues related to sex and adopts a moralistic stance in dealing with sex work, homosexuality and drug use. Hence there is an unwillingness to discuss and engage with core elements driving the epidemic. This hampers the collection of needed data and effective preventive action.

In the health sector, as in other sectors, allocation of resources depends on the relative power of different social groups. The prevalence of HIV is disproportionately higher among the weaker socio-economic groups. Hence issues related to HIV receive less attention, especially since the needed strategies are not easy to support. Due to the same reason, the quality of human resources the programme attracts too suffers in comparison to other areas.

Politics of international health

To some extent the differentials in lack of power of major beneficiaries of AIDS control programme is counteracted by the priority assigned to HIV by international donors. Allocation of global resources is determined by preferences of decision makers in donor countries. This will be dictated by the perceived interests of the population of these countries. HIV, a disease which has had its impact in the developed world, which is yet to be medically managed through effective vaccine or drugs and whose ability to mutate is not fully mapped, is perceived as threatening by the donor countries. Hence it suits both altruistic and selfish motives of the donors to allocate resources to HIV prevention and research. The affected and infected population in the developed world have organised themselves to function as a pressure group. Such pressures have influenced both the structure of the programme and allocation of resources. They have also been able to support the growth of similar organisations in India whose impact is being felt in the decision-making in the country.

The current structures

The implementation of National AIDS Prevention and Control Programmes is led by the National AIDS Control Organisation (NACO). It was constituted as the National AIDS Committee in 1986 to facilitate the initiation of National AIDS Control Programme

(NACP) in 1987. In 1992, the Government of India re-formed the organisation into the NACO within the Ministry of Health. Its activities are funded by national government and donor funds. There are other players who operate without linking up with the national programme. The government programme is led in states by the State AIDS Control Societies (SACS). Non-government implementers have either state management institutions or state-level partners. Some donors also have funds that operate independent of NACO. A few donors fund states directly.

National and state level structures

National AIDS Control Organisation is an integral part of the ministry of health, headed by a senior official of the ministry (implementation arrangements of NACP follows NACO 1999a). It has three oversight bodies: one headed by Secretary (Health), Government of India and another by the Minister of Health and the National Council on AIDS, headed by the Prime Minister. It is governed by all Government of India regulations and accountability systems such as Comptroller and Auditor General and Parliamentary oversight. While this reduces the flexibility of management, it also supports implementation of the programme with the prestige of being a government department. Being located in health department, it is strong on health related interventions but is hamstrung when dealing with other sectors whose contribution is vital to the control of AIDS epidemic.

During the first phase of World Bank funded National AIDS Control Programme, State AIDS Cells were set up in departments of health in state governments to manage state level interventions. The AIDS Cells could not break free of the managerial and fiscal constraints of operating within the health department. Consequently, much of the non-health elements of the AIDS Control programme did not get implemented in most parts of the country. When the programme was scaled up in the second phase in 1999, state structures were reorganised as SACS with a fair degree of autonomy and substantially scaled up staffing.

However, a corresponding increase of staff did not take place in NACO. Senior officials of the organisation were on deputation from different cadres of the Government of India and were not selected based on qualification and experience. The resultant gap in technical expertise was made good with the help of consultants supported by development partners. This created disconnect in technical oversight with the authority and skills being vested at different points. While the support of consultants enabled the organisation to meet its immediate needs, it did not create the institutional learning and memory to adapt the organisation to the needs of a dynamic epidemic. It also created a situation where some of the peripheral units (NGOs, SACS) which made use of the autonomy granted to them had skills superior to the central unit. But in some states, interventions under the first and second phase hardly took off.

The Human resources needed at NACO and SACS has to cover social sector and health related skills, in addition to the staff functions. The contribution of non-medical factors to good health had been officially recognised since the Alma Ata Declaration, but given the stranglehold of the professional monopolists of the medical profession over national and international health bodies, services other than biomedical ones were given very little importance even in such areas as maternal and child health and mental health. But since non-medical personnel had established themselves in AIDS response, programme managers have had to reconcile the claims of non-biomedical responses such as counselling, motivation to adopt and sustain safe behaviours and provision of information. The tension between the two sets of service providers may have hampered the integration of HIV into health services. But it has also led to the adoption of essential non-medical elements to the response which has been kept out of other programmes. In comparison to other public health programmes, AIDS control has seen much higher levels of civil society participation. But the developments in diagnostics and treatment may gradually ensure medicalisation of this programme too.

Managing collaborating partners

Successful prevention and treatment programmes are not possible without the support of other sector ministries, private sector
and NGOs. Sectors that employ a large number of persons such
as Railways, Coal and Mines, Steel and uniformed services can
make a major difference to prevention if they mainstream HIV
into their functioning. Private sector, especially in health care,
will need to supplement government efforts in treatment. Since
most of the behaviours that contribute to the spread of HIV are
illegal or not socially acceptable, they cannot be reached by
government structures. Non-government or community-based
organisations have the required skills and flexibility to reach
such hard to reach subpopulations. Hence the support of many
partners is necessary for a successful HIV prevention and control
programme. Programme managers need to be skilled in managing such collaborations.

Linkages to other implementing agencies

Global interest and availability of funding has seen the emergence
of a large number of agencies to implement AIDS prevention
and control programmes. There is no mechanism to ensure that
all players act on the same script. Since this is an international
phenomenon, the donor agencies, led by UNAIDS, had agreed
on the 'Three ones' principles to which all donor agencies are
signatories (UNAIDS 2004). One of the principles to ensure coordination (in addition to one commonly agreed framework and
a common monitoring and evaluation system) is to have 'One
National AIDS Coordinating Authority with a broad based
multi-sector mandate'. If NACO is to function as the national
authority coordinating AIDS control activities, its structure needs
to become more broad based and systems for coordination, including developing one common plan covering all agencies at
the national and state levels, have to be put in place. In a country
like India, this is best done at the district level. But the centralised nature of the NACP and most of the donor-funded programmes make such an alignment unlikely at the district level.
However, aligning all programmes irrespective of who implements
them is necessary to optimise the use of resources and to prevent

wasteful duplication. The needed systems are yet to be developed and vested interests may ensure that this never happens.

Technical support

AIDS Control Programme is relatively new. It has elements which require different combination of skills. The need for providing technical support to ensure quality in prevention and treatment programmes was recognised when the second phase was designed. National institutions of excellence were identified to function as Technical Resource Groups where capacities would be available or built up (NACO 1999a). National AIDS Control Organisation, State AIDS Control Society (SACS) and other implementing partners were to access technical support from these institutions. But due to faulty design and shortage of funds, these institutions did not become functional. Hence implementing agencies did not have access to the needed technical support, with implications for quality. Technical support was available only in states with bilateral support. Most of them profited from it and the impact was seen in the quality of their response.

However to make a difference to the epidemic, technical programming in the highly vulnerable states of North India has to improve. One option that will be tried out is to replicate the Technical Support Units (TSUs) that functioned well in South and West India. But the experience of Orissa, which had access to a TSU but did not have the skill to manage the technical support, shows that if the quality of management of SACS is weak, the presence of a TSU may not make a crucial difference. And the standard SACS in states with weak governance structures are not likely to improve in a hurry. So NACO has to develop innovative strategies like performance based funding and direct collaboration with implementing partners. NACO also needs to wean foundations and donors who can adopt more flexible strategies away from states where conditions for success are better (where they would prefer to work) towards states and areas where the need is greater.

Structures to address an evolving epidemic

While the predicted Armageddon has not come to pass in India, problems associated with HIV/AIDS has continued to grow and diversify, with the response barely keeping pace. In the new phase of AIDS control programme slated to start from early 2007, there will be a coordinated effort to scale up the response. Since the epidemic has matured, there will be greater emphasis on treatment and impact mitigation requiring more human and financial resources. This is expected to be made available partly through additional investments in public sector and partly through public-private partnerships.

National AIDS Control Organisation and SACS will be strengthened to deal with newer and larger programmes, but since government rules prohibit staff expansion on a large scale, many functions will have to be out-sourced. Contract management, in which health sector has been notoriously weak (Nandraj et al. 2001), will be an important component of the AIDS control programme. For greater decentralisation, implementing arrangements will also be set up at the district level.

Efforts will be made to institutionalise evidence based planning and management and technical support. Strategic information units, which analyse data and generate information for decision makers, will be set up in all state and national units. All the major states will have access to the services of a TSU. Training will be overseen by a multidisciplinary committee at the national level and conducted by national and regional centres of excellence. There will be special arrangements to support the implementation of the programme in weaker states, even though the precise nature of such arrangements is not clear yet.

Challenges in implementing AIDS control programme

While the AIDS control programme is subject to problems common to all centrally sponsored schemes (straitjacketed design and implementation arrangements, lack of ownership by implementing units and lack of clarity of accountability between centre and peripheral units), its management is further complicated by some challenges specific to HIV/AIDS.

Stigma of the drivers of the epidemic

HIV affects some sub-populations more than others due to their occupation, sexual preferences or recreational habits (Plummer et al. 1991). Low socio-economic status and gender disparities also increase vulnerabilities. The thrust of AIDS prevention activities has been to reduce the risk of infection among these highly vulnerable sub-populations. But many of their practises—sex work, homosexuality and injecting drug use—are punishable under the law and frowned upon by the society. These sub-populations are generally not organised and not willing to deal with government agencies. SACS have the difficult task of convincing vulnerable populations to cooperate, persuading them to adopt practices which are not easy on a sustained basis, neutralising structural constraints that add to their vulnerability and ensuring that other government agencies, such as the criminal justice system, do not undo their work by persecuting their partners in prevention. To tide over this difficulty, NGOs are contracted to manage the interface with vulnerable communities.

This raises a series of governance issues. SACS are often not in a position to protect their partners in a government sponsored programme from opposition from other government agencies which are also implementing the laws approved by Parliament. The only way to remove this paradox is to amend laws that inhibit prevention activities. This goes against median social values and legislators will be unwilling to support the measure in near future. But in some states where good NGOs have been working, their competence has ensured that their work with vulnerable communities have transcended these limitations and they have persuaded these communities to adopt safer behaviours.

There are no implementing structures below the State AIDS Control Society level for the AIDS control programme. The implementation machinery is the health department. Due to the stigma associated with the disease, health departments had been unwilling, with honourable exceptions, to provide even the biomedical contribution to the control of the epidemic. As familiarity with the disease grows and competence is built up, ownership by health department is likely to grow. In time, the need to deal with the epidemic may have the consequence of decriminalising many of the activities currently frowned upon.

Mainstreaming with other sectors

Many of the factors that drive the AIDS epidemic lie outside the zone of influence of the health sector. This includes such factors as migration, poverty, illiteracy and disempowerment. Neither the health sector nor AIDS control activists have the reach needed to control an epidemic that has spread to the general population. This can be managed only if HIV is mainstreamed into the functioning of other sectors. Managers in these sectors need to be convinced to take steps to protect their employees and clients from the epidemic and make the changes needed to slow down the factors spreading the epidemic. But since HIV is perceived as the problem of one sector alone, managers in other sectors do not have the incentive to perform these functions. We need systems and a change of attitude among both AIDS programmes managers and managers of the concerned sectors to facilitate such cooperation.

Coordination with other health programmes

Even within the health sector, HIV has functioned in a stand alone fashion. It has not been able to exploit the synergies that exist with other health related programmes, such as reproductive health, TB control and mental health. This has opportunity costs for all related programmes. The coordination arrangements envisaged under the National Rural Health Mission (NRHM) may solve some of these. But the dynamics of AIDS Control working with the national, state and district level structures of NRHM are yet to be worked out.

Integration of different AIDS programmes

Due to the high priority accorded to it by international donor agencies, AIDS programmes have seen a windfall of funding in recent years. However, the absence of a common agreed upon strategic plan has led to over allocation of funds to some regions, duplication of projects, poor dovetailing of projects and gaps in funding. This is an international phenomenon. In order to counter it, the international donor community, led by the UN, has laid down the 'Principle of Three Ones': one agreed national framework led by the national leadership that is the basis for coordinating the work of all partners; one National AIDS Coordinating Authority, with a broad based multi-sector mandate and one agreed country level Monitoring and Evaluation System. Such a programme has to emerge in India too. But a government managed programme has the danger of deteriorating into a government dictated programme. This will take away the flexibility that many implementing partners enjoy and its implications for programming may not be salutary. Systems have to be deployed so that national management structures become more participatory and partners are able to sign into them without being choked in government diktats.

A similar tension between the need for integration and flexibility for innovation also exists in the NGO-funded part of the national programme. NGOs are engaged so that they can bring greater flexibility to the programme. But having accepted funds from the consolidated fund of India, they become answerable to all the checks and balances that government agencies are subjected to, making a mockery of the flexibility for which they were hired in the first place.

Differentials in response scale and quality between states

As in the most development programmes of India, states differ in the extent and quality of implementation of AIDS control programmes. Most disease control programmes do well in the southern and western states. Other states too catch up till a large reservoir is left in the Hindi speaking belt. HIV shows no sign of being an exception. But if our experience of small pox and polio eradication is any indication and if the epidemic is allowed to take root, the resources that the country would have to spend on reversing the epidemic in these states will be very high. It makes sense to front load prevention efforts in these states so as to avoid a full blown epidemic. But these states have been extremely laggard in prevention efforts. The ability of national programme managers to intervene is also constrained by the federal system. Unless this is sorted out at the political and bureaucratic levels, differentials in AIDS epidemic may come to resemble other disease burden: managed in some states, rampant in others. Considering the population and vulnerabilities of the underperforming states, this is a scary scenario. The problems posed by the epidemic in the conflict ridden parts of north east pose another major challenge.

Higher order programming

AIDS is not only a recent epidemic but also a rapidly evolving one. This leads to fresh challenges which require higher skills to manage. For instance, the supply driven prevention programmes among vulnerable populations, after initial successes, are likely to plateau unless other needs and constraints that come up are addressed. If first generation anti retrovirals are widely available, the need for more efficient management of side effects and resistance would emerge. Since some resistance is certain, there will be an increasing demand for next generation drugs. Putting persons on ARV also leads to the need for support systems to ensure treatment compliance and access to livelihood. As parents get affected, the needs of orphans need to be addressed by the government. Non-Governmental Organisations and community organisations who are the primary managers dealing with the problems on the field are the ones who can best develop solutions to emerging problems. However, there are no learning systems and therefore, the experience of NGOs can be a feedback into the official programme.

Generating and accessing technical support including human resources

AIDS control programmes call for a wide variety of technical skills. These include the ability to work with vulnerable populations, combine demand generation with provision of services to unreached populations and reconcile the demands of respecting privacy with collecting the needed information and effecting changes in private behaviours. Many of these would have to be learned in the field. Given the urgency of scaling up the response in regions with the worst structures for development of human resources, innovative systems need to be developed to make the needed human resources available. At present there are no systems for horizontal learning between states and other implementing partners. Increased funding for HIV programmes will also make it difficult to retain good personnel in government programmes. The shortage of competent persons may emerge as a constraint in future unless human resource needs are planned for.

Use of strategic information for planning and midcourse correction

Programme managers in India rarely make use of data and analysis for programme design and management. In other programmes this is made good by past experience of managers in the sector. Many of them have managed the programme at different levels. Senior programme managers who manage HIV programmes are often first time entrants to the HIV field. Since they are not familiar with the programme, they focus on familiar areas, such as control of blood borne infections. This may not be the optimal strategy to control the epidemic. Unless programme managers have access to reliable data and are trained to base their activities on the results of the analysis of this information, the quality of HIV programming will be low and stress will continue on components with higher comfort levels, not on those which best impact the epidemic. Without good systems for collection and analysis of data, this fact would not even be comprehended by managers.

Conclusion

It is true that HIV has common features with many other public health programmes. However, it has some unique attributes. This is due in part to the epidemiology of the disease and in part to the history of the epidemic. Some of the positive aspects AIDS has brought about, such as greater involvement of civil society organisation, support for mobilisation of infected persons

and insistence on respect for human rights have the potential
to transform practices in other health fields. Since there is an
urgent need for an effective response and since the response
cannot be effective without addressing some very contentious
issues, HIV has created an opportunity and a compulsion to be
innovative in dealing with them. It has also opened up challenges
for programme managers. The history of implementation of
the AIDS control programme in some parts of the nation shows
that India has the ability to deal with the challenges. If this can
be generalised to all Indian states and programme managers
are willing to learn and adapt from their experience, India will
be able to keep the epidemic and its impact at a minimum, much
lower than the bleak scenario predicted for the country by the
foretellers of doom.

References

Kumar, R., P. Jha, P. Arora, P. Mony, P. Bhatia, P. Millson, N. Dhingra,
M. Bhattacharya, R. S. Remis and N. Nagelkerke. 2006. 'Trends
in HIV-1 in Young Adults in South India from 2000 to 2004: A
Prevalence Study', *Lancet*, 367 (9517): 1164–72.

Nandraj, Sunil, V. R. Muraleedharan, Rama, Baru, Imrana, Quadeer
and Ritu Priya. 2001. 'Private Health Sector in India'. Chennai: IIT,
New Delhi: JNU, February 2001.

National AIDS Control Organisation (NACO). 1999a. *Scheme for the
Prevention and Control of AIDS*. New Delhi: Ministry of Health and
Family Welfare, Government of India.

———. 1999b. *Project Implementation Plan for National AIDS Control
Project Phase II (1999–2004)*. New Delhi: Ministry of Health and
Family Welfare, Government of India.

Plummer, F. A., N. J. Nagelkerke, S. Moses, J. O. Ndinya-Achola,
J. Bwayo and E. Ngugi. 1991. 'The Importance of Core Groups in
the Epidemiology and Control of HIV-1 Infection' AIDS; 5 (Suppl 1)
169–76.

UNAIDS. 2004. '"Three Ones" key principles: Coordination of Na-
tional Responses to HIV/AIDS—Guiding Principles for National
Authorities and Their Partners', Conference Paper No. 1, Washington
Consultation on 'Three ones', Geneva.

———. 2006. *Report on the Global Epidemic*. Geneva: Joint UN Programme on HIV/AIDS.

National Rural Health Mission: A Brief Introduction

13

DILEEP MAVALANKAR

Background

The United Progressive Alliance (UPA) government elected to power in May 2004 promised to increase government health expenditure from 1 per cent of the GDP to 2–3 per cent. This was a major political commitment to reversing the decline in public expenditure on health by India that had been occurring over the last several years. To implement this major investment in health, the Union Cabinet approved the Ministry of Health and Family Welfare's proposal on 4 January 2005 to set up a special programme called the National Rural Health Mission (NRHM) that would extend from 2005–12. In India, the word 'mission' is used for a high-powered special programme generally backed by a high level of political commitment to achieve specific developmental objectives in a rapid and time-bound manner. For example, in the past there has been a telecom mission which helped spread availability of telecommunication in rural areas. NRHM was to have a preparatory phase from January to March 2005, during which the basic design of the programme was developed. NRHM was officially launched by the Prime Minister on 12 April 2005.

The vision of NRHM

The vision of NRHM is broad and includes the following:

1. Architectural correction in health care delivery.
2. Special focus on 18 states with weak indicators.
3. Improving the availability of quality health care in rural areas.
4. Creating synergy between health and determinants of good health.
5. Mainstreaming the Indian systems of medicine.
6. Building capacity.
7. Involving the community in the planning process.

Thus, NRHM seems to change many of the basic structures and systems of health care and move it towards a much broader overall improvement in health, rather than just focussing on reproductive and child health.

Outcomes to be achieved by NRHM by 2012

NRHM has set very specific and ambitious outcome targets for maternal and child health improvement, fertility reduction and disease control. These are as follows:

1. IMR reduced to 30/1,000 live births by 2012.
2. MMR reduced to 100/100,000 live births by 2012.
3. TFR reduced to 2.1 by 2012.
4. Malaria Mortality Reduction Rate—60 per cent by 2012.
5. Kala Azar eliminated by 2010.
6. Filaria reduced by 80 per cent by 2010.
7. Dengue Mortality reduced by 50 per cent by 2012.
8. Leprosy eliminated by December 2005.
9. TB DOTS—maintain 85 per cent cure rate.

It can be seen from the above indicators that for at least some of them, there is no reliable measurement system, for example,

Maternal Mortality Reduction (MMR), malaria and dengue mortality. We hope that under NRHM, such systems will be developed.

NRHM—the concept

The key concept in NRHM is to bring all the health and family welfare programmes, including reproductive and child health (RCH-II), under one umbrella. Thus, in effect, merging of the health and family welfare divisions of the Government of India is a major policy and structural change. Determinants of health like nutrition, sanitation and drinking water supply are also to be addressed under NRHM, perhaps through close coordination with sister departments and ministries that deal with these subjects.

Core strategies

The overall objectives of NRHM are to be achieved through six core strategies, which are, establishing community health workers called ASHA, infrastructure improvements, capacity building, private-public partnership, risk pooling and social health insurance and decentralised planning. The indicative details of these are given further:

Community health worker (ASHA)

'ASHA' is an acronym that stands for Accredited Social Health Activist. The Hindi meaning of 'ASHA' is hope. It is evident that NRHM has put a lot of emphasis and effort into community health workers. ASHAs will be chosen by and accountable to the panchayat and will work as a link between the community and the health delivery system. They will be volunteers but will receive performance-linked incentives for promotion of universal immunisation, referral and escort services for mothers. ASHAs will work closely with the Integrated Child Development Scheme (ICDS) programme and will be anchored in the Anganwadi system. They will also have some curative responsibility to treat common illnesses at the village level and hence they will be given a basic drug kit and act as a depot holder for contraceptives and Information Education and Communication (IEC) materials. Thus, ASHA is a new and revised version of the 'village health worker' idea that was originally tried in India in 1977 but did not succeed due to lack of support.

Infrastructure improvement

NRHM's second key strategy is to strengthen existing health infrastructure. The major component of infrastructural improvement will be revision of population norms for sub-centres. Provision of untied funds for each sub-centre will be Rs 10,000 per annum for various activities, including minor repairs, innovation and other expenditure for facilitating work. The next level of improvement is to make 50 per cent of Public Health Centres (PHCs) operational on a 24-hour, 7-day-a-week basis for provision of delivery and other basic emergency services. Additionally, all Community Health Centres (CHCs) are to be operational as First Referral Units (FRUs), providing emergency obstetric and newborn care. At the district level, one Mobile Medical Unit is to be available for providing care to difficult-to-reach areas.

As part of NRHM, the government is developing norms for the infrastructure, staff, equipment and management of public health facilities; these are called Indian Public Health Standards (IPHS). The first draft of IPHS has been developed for CHCs and is being circulated. Committees of stakeholders, called 'Rogi Kalyan Samitis', are to be formed and promoted for each level of health facilities. The key role of these will be the cost recovery and stakeholder participation in the management of health facilities.

NRHM also wants to mainstream 'AYUSH', which is an acronym for Indian and traditional systems of medicine in Government health facilities. NRHM aims to introduce mainstreaming of AYUSH into the private sector.

The supply of essential drugs, both allopathic and AYUSH, to sub-centres, PHCs and CHCs is one of the key strategies of NRHM for improving service delivery in the government facility.

Capacity building

NRHM lays great stress on building capacity throughout various levels in the health system, with special focus on support services such as financial and accounting services. These will become more professionalised by introducing professionals such as MBAs and Chartered Accountants at both district and state levels. NRHM will also induct Skilled Mission Teams at each level.

Comprehensive training will be arranged for all categories of staff, and even members of Panchayati Raj Institutions (PRIs) will receive training to improve their role in health programmes. ASHAs will receive appropriate training and will be supported by a mentoring group formed from various reputed non-governmental organisations (NGOs), academics and government officers.

Public-private partnership

Public-private partnerships PPP will be one of the most import-ant strategies for improving service delivery. The government seems to recognise that it alone cannot provide all health services and that the private sector has an important role to play, and so NRHM will develop guidelines for accreditation of private health providers. Pilots on social franchising and contracting in selected districts will be developed to learn from them, and then subsequently scaled up to larger areas.

Risk pooling and social health insurance

NRHM recognises the importance of risk pooling and social health insurance, as this will be a good way of providing health service financing. A Task Group is currently working on these aspects and will provide a report soon. Pilot test will be started in different parts of the country, and lessons learned from implementation of these pilots will guide the strategy of risk pooling and social health insurance under NRHM.

Decentralised planning

NRHM assigns great importance to decentralised planning and thus is a major departure from the previous family welfare programme, which was highly centralised and target oriented. NRHM will provide a financial envelope to districts on normative basis and districts will be given the freedom to select the interventions more suitable for that area. The states and districts will be encouraged to prepare perspective planning as well as annual plans, and a small component will be set aside for state- and district-level innovations. The states will be encouraged to involve the community and PRIs in developing the village and district Health Plans. This bottom-up planning process should lead to district plans that will converge into one state plan. NRHM will help strengthen state and district planning and appraisal capacities.

Institutional framework

The institutional framework of NRHM will consist of a high-powered National Steering group, below which a Mission Steering group will be constituted. For important decisions, an empowered programme committee will be formed. These three bodies will be composed of elected representatives of citizens, government officers, NGOs and selected academic experts and these bodies will guide the mission's directorate. At the central level, the Mission Directorate will be headed by an Additional Secretary. Each state will constitute the State Health Mission with a merger of all the state health societies. At the facility level, the district health mission will form a 'Rogi Kalyan Samiti' to support the health facilities. At the village level, village health committees will be activated.

District health plan

Under NRHM, the district becomes the core unit of planning, budgeting and implementation and the District Health Plan will be a basic building block for health planning. The District Health Plan will be based on an amalgamation of field responses from village and block health plans, and will take into account and integrate state level and national priorities for health, water supply, sanitation and nutrition. This will increase the effectiveness of health services and blocks, in turn, will be strengthened to develop their own plan based on local needs.

All health related societies at the district level will be merged into one common 'District Health Mission', and similarly, all state level health related societies will merge into one State Health Mission.

Each district will have a project management unit to strengthen the management capacities at the district level. Similarly, the states will have project management units.

Action points at district level

NRHM envisages the following action points for specific and quick implementation of the overall strategy:

1. Constitution of District Health Mission.
2. Preparation of an Integrated District Health Plan.
3. Preparation of Village & Block Health Plan(s).
4. Integration of ICDS, Total Sanitation Campaign & Health.
5. Constitution of Quality Assurance Committee(s).
6. Training, Organisation and Integration of Project Management Units (PMUs).
7. Increasing participation of PRIs.
8. Constitution of Rogi Kalyan Samiti(s).
9. Partnership(s) with NGOs, Private Health Facilities and Professional Medical Associations.
10. Strengthening of Immunisation Programmes.
11. Operationalisation of the Janani Suraksha Yojana (JSY) scheme.

The states have been instructed to take rapid action in this direction.

Action points at district level for JSY

NRHM envisages following action points at the district level for JSY:

1. Make Sub-centres and Anganwadis effective meeting points for women.
2. Simplify procedures for Below Poverty Line (BPL) certification.
3. Operationalise 24/7 delivery services at the PHC/CHC levels for provision of basic obstetric care.

4. Create partnerships with private health sector institutions through reorganisation/accreditation processes for provision of obstetric services to JSY beneficiaries.
5. Placing advance cash with Auxiliary Nurse Midwives (ANMs)/ASHAs.

Action points at district level for immunisation

NRHM has developed the following specific action points to improve immunisation services at the district level:

1. Dedicate a District Immunisation Officer as programme manager.
2. Strengthen the 'fixed day and fixed time' strategy.
3. Micro-plans to be made.
4. Improve transport and distribution plan of vaccines.
5. Ensure that vaccine vans are in working condition.
6. Timely flow of funds.
7. Improve cold-chain maintenance.
8. Develop plans for alternate vaccine delivery.
9. Increase availability of ANMs at the session site.
10. Assign alternate service providers.

Role of states

Under NRHM, specific points are identified where states must take prompt action. These are as follows:

1. Develop a constitution for the State Health Mission.
2. Integrate Health and Family Welfare Societies.
3. Prepare an integrated NRHM State Action Plan.
4. Merge the Departments of Health and Family Welfare.
5. Enter into MoU with Government of India.
6. Involve PRIs.
7. Strengthen PMUs.
8. Finalise state models for ASHA, including remuneration package.
9. Initiate selection of at least 40 per cent ASHAs in first year.
10. Finalise training modules and initiate trainings.

Role of state infrastructure

NRHM envisages that states will undertake special efforts to improve the conditions and increase the utilisation of health infrastructure. The states are requested to identify two CHCs per district for up-gradation during the first year; select agencies for the construction and procurement of equipment; develop a timeframe for upgrading health facilities; set up a mechanism for procurement and logistic issues; develop a plan for mainstreaming AYUSH; and ensure performance benchmarking of institutions. Additionally, if needed, district cadres of doctors and block cadres of ANMs will be formed and availability of doctors in rural areas will be ensured through the pooling concept at the block level. Last, a model for Public-Private Partnership in health will be developed.

Key activities accomplished

Given the high level of political commitment, starting with the Prime Minister's Secretariat, NRHM strategies and activities have taken rapid strides. In the past year and half, since its formation, a lot of preparatory work and progress has been made. NRHM has established an institutional framework including the Mission Steering Group, Empowered Programme Committee, Mission Directorate, Advisory Group on Community Action, Committee on Inter-sectoral Convergence, National Programme Coordination Committee, North East Advisory Committee and Mentoring Group for ASHA.

Guidelines disseminated

NRHM has produced various guidelines and documents, including the following:

1. Mission Document
2. IPHS
3. ASHA—introductory documents
4. Training module for ASHA
5. State Health Mission/District Health Mission

6. Merger of Societies
7. Draft MoU for states
8. Skilled Birth Attendants

Untied funds to sub-centers

Money has been released to states for untied grants of Rs 10,000 per sub-centre to be spent in supervisor of Panchayats.

Up-gradation and strengthening of CHCs/PHCs

States were asked to identify two CHCs per district for up-gradation. As a first installment, Rs 2 million for each CHC was released to the states, and a second installment will be released after facility surveys are completed. IPHS guidelines for PHCs/sub-centres are being drafted.

Capacity building

Induction of 700 professionals—including MBAs and Chartered Accountants—will be done at both state and district levels in PMUs in the EAG states. These professionals have already started working in many states. Rs 1 million per district was released in 50 per cent of the EAG states for district planning.

Stepping up of immunisation

Activities for strengthening immunisation programmes are underway. This process includes introduction of AD Syringes, development of alternate vaccine delivery systems, and provision of mobility support to districts and states for supervision and support for the cold chain.

Increased focus on financial management

The newly inducted professionals are helping to improve financial management at the state and district levels. This has resulted in a reduction of pending utilisation certificates from Rs 61.3 billion in March 2004 to Rs 36.3 billion in July 2005, and the unspent balance was reduced by Rs 9 billion in the last 6 months.

New TASK GROUPS formed

To gather inputs from various experts, NGOs and field level people, the Government of India formed various task groups regarding the goals for the development of various guidelines, documents and strategies. These included PHS, the role of PRIs, ASHA, technical support for NRHM, public-private partnership, urban health mission, medical education, risk pooling/health insurance, as well as task groups on health financing mechanisms and guidelines for district action plans. Many of these groups have already submitted their reports.

Other activities accomplished

Many states have already merged their Departments of Health and Family Welfare, launched both the RCH II and JSY programmes and set up Mother Non-Government Organisation (MNGOs) in 314 Districts. The family welfare linked health insurance scheme is ready, with special attention to the north eastern states, and a Regional Resource Centre has been established at Guwahati.

Table 13.1   Activities accomplished under NRHM at state level

Activities	No. of states
NRHM formally Launched	7
State Health Mission Formed	20
Constitution of District Health Mission	14
Merger of Departments of Health and Family Welfare	19
Merger of Societies at State and District level	14
Formation of Rogi Kalyan Samiti	16
Finalisation of ASHA Model	4
Action Plan for mainstreaming AYUSH	5
Number of MNGOs set up	209

Source: The presentation on National Rural Health Mission (NRHM) sent by Mrs Jalaja, Additional Secretary, NRHM, Government of India, New Delhi.

Conclusion

This chapter has outlined the vision, concept, core strategies and activities designated under NRHM. It shows that with a high level of political commitment, substantial changes were initiated in the health and family welfare departments of both the central and state governments. If this tempo of implementation continues with proper guidance, monitoring and adequate resources, it seems that NRHM has real potential to bring about substantial improvement in rural health services in India. If NRHM succeeds in its strategies, then by 2012, substantial improvements in health infrastructure and health conditions in India are likely. The success of NRHM depends large on political commitment, administrative acumen and technical-evidence-based direction.

Acknowledgement

This is a paper based on a presentation on National Rural Health Mission (NRHM) sent by Mrs Jalaja, Additional Secretary, NRHM, Government of India, New Delhi.

Achieving the Millennium Development Goals for Maternal and Newborn Health

14

ARDI KAPTININGSIH

Introduction

Adopted in the year 2000, the United Nations Millennium Development Goals (MDGs) seek to address key issues in world-wide development by setting specific targets for the reduction of poverty, morbidity, mortality and gender inequality by 2015. MDG-5 aims to reduce the MMR (measles, mumps and rubella) by three quarters from its level in 1990. One of its measures is to increase the proportion of births attended by skilled health personnel to at least 50 per cent in 2010 and 60 per cent in 2015 for high MMR countries, and universal skilled care at birth globally. The objective of MDG-4 is to achieve an under-five mortality rate reduction by two thirds, which would require reduction of neonatal mortality rate by 50 per cent.

The South-East Asia Region (SEAR) accounts for approximately 174,000 maternal and 1.4 million neonatal deaths every year, which shares 33 and 35 per cent of global figures, respectively. Most complications responsible for maternal and neonatal mortality occur during childbirth and immediate postpartum period. Therefore, timely access to 'skilled care at birth' is often the most critical factor for the survival of women and their newborns. At the primary level, skilled care should be provided by health personnel with midwifery skills (skilled attendants), while complications at the secondary level require health personnel with obstetric, anaesthetic and paediatric skills.

Countries with low maternal and neonatal mortality rates have higher access to skilled care at birth. This demonstrates that skilled care at birth is an essential aspect during delivery and the immediate post-partum period. This care includes routine or normal treatment, management of obstetric complications and any necessary special attention. A skilled midwife—with proper equipment, supplies and drugs—is crucial for maternal care at primary care level. In case of emergency, a referral system with proper transportation, cost subsidies and effective communication channels becomes critical. Elements of skilled birth care at the second level require a hospital with basic facilities; the right personnel, including an obstetrician, paediatrician and anaesthesiologist; and accessible supplies such as equipment, drugs and safe blood (see Figure 14.1).

Figure 14.1 Elements of skilled care at birth

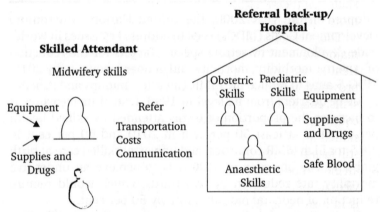

Source: SEARO.

Scenario-based challenges in SEAR countries

Countries in the SEAR are at different stages of development of skilled care at birth. In Bangladesh, Bhutan, India, Nepal and Timor-Leste, less than 50 per cent of the births are attended by skilled attendants. The effect of skilled birth attendance can be easily observed while comparing data on maternal and neonatal mortality in SEAR countries (Table 14.1). Thailand, DPR Korea and Sri Lanka had the lowest maternal mortality ratio and neonatal mortality rate, with the highest proportion of births attended by skilled health personnel. The key issues contributing to this success are high-levels of political commitment, development of long-term strategic plans, promotion of community-based midwifery care, and lastly, establishing and maintaining functioning health systems that provide regulation of skilled attendants with an effective monitoring system.

In Indonesia, there has been an expansion of accredited midwifery-trained health staff for skilled care at birth while establishing partnerships between skilled attendants and traditional birth attendants. In Bangladesh, there is short-term midwifery training for existing health staffs for the improvement of their skills. On the other hand, in India, the government aims to promote facility-based childbirth.

The lack of skilled attendants at the community level is a major concern affecting the low level of skilled care at birth. Health care providers are not able to fulfil their responsibility of providing maternal and newborn care due to a lack of essential skills, equipment, support networks and/or referral services. Few countries have succeeded in deploying an adequate number of skilled attendants at the community level, but those that have still face various other challenges. These countries need to ensure all elements of skilled care at birth include proper outreach services for poor and disadvantaged groups. An additional challenge is in instituting adequate and appropriate career development schemes that will ensure retention of standards of maternal and newborn health service throughout communities. Countries with high coverage of skilled care at birth may still have areas with poor access, and such countries often face problems related to overuse of ultrasound screening and a high rate of caesarean sections.

While looking at the challenges facing SEAR countries, the above discussion shows that there are competing priorities to improve access and quality of care for those countries with less than 50 per cent of births attended by skilled attendants. Few countries

Table 14.1 Selected maternal and neonatal health indicators, 2000

No	Country	No. of maternal deaths	Maternal mortality ratio (per 100,000 live births)	No. of neonatal deaths	Neonatal mortality rate (per 1,000 live births)	Proportion (%) of births attended by skilled health personnel in 2002
1	Bangladesh	16,000	380	163,800	39	21.8
2	Bhutan	310	420	2,380	34	23.7
3	DPR Korea	260	67	7,020	18	98.6
4	India	136,000	540	1,058,400	42	42.3
5	Indonesia	10,000	230	94,500	21	68.4
6	Maldives	10	110	290	29	70.3
7	Myanmar	4,300	360	44,400	37	77.5
8	Nepal	6,000	740	35,640	44	13.0
9	Sri Lanka	300	92	3,960	12	97.0
10	Thailand	520	44	19,200	16	94.5
11	Timor-Leste	140	660	n.a	n.a	19.5
	Total	**173,840**		**1,429,590**		

with a medium level of attendance—between 50 and 80 per cent of births—need to strengthen logistical and referral systems and improve quality of care. On the contrary, in countries with a very high success rate—attendance at greater than 80 per cent of births—it becomes necessary to determine which areas have not been reached by services and to reduce the over-medicalisation of normal pregnancy and childbirth.

Policy and key issues

Certain policy issues are crucial for those countries with a low proportion of deliveries by skilled attendants, that is, human resources for maternal and newborn health. The right policy would ensure availability of skilled attendants with appropriate midwifery skills at primary health care level. However, this needs a referral back up system that provides emergency obstetric care and special care for newborns, and the proper delegation of authority within a functioning health system.

Human resource development and management are crucial issues, just as availability of a sufficient number of skilled birth attendants at the community level is essential for achieving high levels of skilled care. Pre-service and in-service training, as well as technical supervision are necessary to increase the quality of services. A key issue involves determining management capacities for the implementation of long-term plans and then establishing proper monitoring and evaluation of these programmes and plans.

Health sector financing is the other key area, which must focus on investments in the health sector. Again, a pro-poor approach should be adopted. Effective and sustainable referral networks must be established between the primary health care level and the first referral units (FRUs). Networking with private institutions, the quality of FRUs, affordable transportation and fair financing mechanisms also need to be considered. Leadership and management need more attention to establish effective and universal skilled attendance at birth, with education being an integral component of developing this. Educating families about positive behaviour change that fosters better practices and thus effective management of community resources is crucial. The other issue relates to multi-sectoral and inter-country collaboration, which encourages government and private sectors, non-profit organisations and community-based organisations to share information, especially related to financing.

Ensuring 'universal access to skilled care at birth' requires a composite of informed, collaborative interventions. Countries must make strategic decisions with long-term vision. The World Health Organisation (WHO) will provide technical support to member states for identifying solutions to these key public health challenges: establishing evidence-based norms and standards for ensuring quality of care, facilitating capacity building, advocating resource mobilisation, and evaluation and monitoring of progress.

References

Bloom S., T. Lippeveld, and D. Wypij, 1999. 'Does Antenatal Care Make a Difference to Safe Delivery? A Study in Urban Uttar Pradesh, India', *Health Policy and Planning*, 14(1): 28–48.

De Bouwere, V., R. Tonglet and Van Lerberghe. 1998. 'Strategies for Reducing Maternal Mortality in Developing Countries: What can we Learn from the History of the Industrialised West?', *Tropical Medicine and International Health*, 3(10): 771–82.

Pathmanathan, I., J. Liljestrand, J. M. Martins, L. C. Rajapaksa, C. Lissner and A. de Silva et al. 2003. Investing in Maternal Health: Learning from Malaysia and Sri Lanka. Washington DC: The World Bank, (Human Development Network, Health, Nutrition and Population Series).

Skilled Care at Every Birth: Report and Documentation of the Technical Discussions held in conjunction with the 42nd Meeting of CCPDM, Dhaka, 5–7 July 2005. World Health Organization, Regional Office for South-East Asia, New Delhi.

Role of Community Participation for Maternal and Child Health: Case Studies from EC Supported Sector Investment Programme in States of Chhattisgarh and Haryana

15

URVASHI CHANDRA
AND SANGEETA SINGH

Introduction

Three goals of any health system in accordance with the World Health Organisation (WHO Report: 2000) are good health, responsiveness to the expectations of the population and fairness of financial contribution. At the Millennium Summit in September 2000, the UN Millennium Declaration was adopted, thereby committing nations to a global partnership for reducing poverty, improving health and promoting peace, human rights, gender equality and environmental sustainability (UN Millennium Development Goals). These themes are also emphasised in the Tenth Five Year Plan (2002–07) of the Government of India (Annex 1).

As described in the report on 'Child Health & Maternal Health' by the Task Force of the UN Millennium Project (Freedman et al. 2005), the state of women and children's health in developing countries continues to be dismal. In case of India, key health indicators are found to be abysmally low.

1. India has one of the highest levels of maternal mortality in the world. Maternal deaths in India account for almost 25 per cent of the world's childbirth-related deaths.
2. Almost half of all children under the age of five are malnourished, and 34 per cent of newborns are underweight.
3. Roughly half the children in the country do not receive complete immunisation.
4. The majority of births in India (58 per cent) are not attended by trained personnel.

A cause for concern is that all over the world, cost-effective, low-tech and simple health interventions do exist, yet the health of women and children, in particular, is appalling nonetheless (Freedman et al. 2005).

For a large majority of people in the South Asian developing countries, the health system appears to be in crisis. A review of the historical development of health systems highlights that these countries were faced with the legacy of colonial health systems that focussed almost exclusively on urban, tertiary hospitals. In order to extend basic curative and preventive measures to rural areas, most countries invested heavily in training and deploying community based health workers. For example, in China, the programme of 'barefoot doctors' was a major success, and in Bangladesh, emphasis was laid on successful strategies such as 'doorstep' family planning services that were designed to circumvent gender based barriers to utilisation (Schuler et al. 1996). It was realised in the early 1960s and 1970s that primary health care is the essential link to any significant improvement in people's health. In 1978, when Mahler proposed 'Health for All', he made it clear that he was referring to the need to provide a level of health that would enable all people, without exception, to live socially and economically productive lives. The Alma Ata Declaration stated that health is a 'fundamental right and the attainment of the highest possible level of health is the most important worldwide social goal whose realisation requires the action of many other social and economic sectors in addition to the health sector'. Furthermore, it stated that primary health care 'forms an integral part both of the country's health system, of which it is the central function and main focus of the overall social and economic development of the community' (Rivero David A. 2003).

Community participation is considered to be one of the cornerstones of most primary health care programmes in the developing world. Also, as mentioned in the Alma Ata declaration, 'People have a right and a duty to participate individually and collectively in the planning and implementation of their health care'. There is ample evidence to show that working with village health workers and community groups at the grassroots level leads to community empowerment, particularly of women.

Role of community in better health services

Most approaches adopted to improve the health of populations use top-down systems, but these have largely been unsuccessful in involving communities. However, community involvement has shown to make health service delivery systems more effective as it builds the community's capacity to identify and address its own health problems.

A community can be defined as 'a group of people with diverse characteristics who are linked by social ties, share common perspectives and engage in joint action in geographical locations or settings' (Macqueen 2001). A community's role is critical for improving health, especially that of mothers and children. The objective of community involvement is to generate awareness and create demand for good quality services. This calls for community mobilisation wherein members are empowered to demand for effective health systems followed by their sustained participation.

Why community participation?

A continuous and interactive process exists between health services and the community availing these services. Therefore, for effective service delivery, community participation is crucial.

Community participation occurs when a community organises itself and takes responsibility for managing its problems. Taking responsibility includes identification of problems, finding solutions, translating them into actions and sustaining changes.

A deliberate strategy of community participation can enhance the process of achievement of better health. This is explained in Figure 15.1.

Figure 15.1 Why community participation?

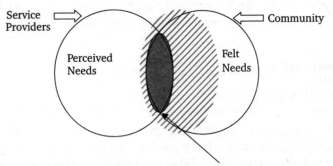

With increasing community participation, this overlap will increase

As represented in Figure 15.1, felt needs are those of the community while perceived needs are as projected by the service providers. At some level, the overlap does exist. However, when the role of the community will increase, more 'felt needs' will be met resulting in greater demand for better health services. If there is a commensurate supply side meeting these needs, there is a likelihood of improved health status of a community.

In essence, some aspects of 'community participation'[1] include:

1. Development of community leaders who effectively disseminate information and correspondingly undertake behavioural reforms to match the 'perceived needs'.
2. A better understanding of the community's 'felt needs', by service providers leading to reforms in service delivery systems. This, in turn, would result in better means to address these felt needs.

3. Equity in planning and management by the community for tackling health issues and bridging the gap between service providers and the community. This will result in greater proximity between the two and is likely to become an effective tool for accountability. This is illustrated in Figure 15.2.

Figure 15.2   Community participation

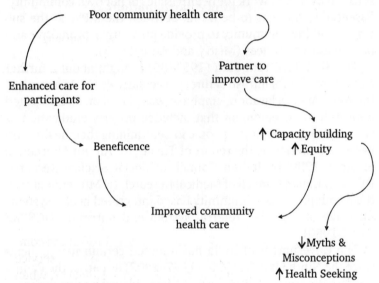

Source: Macqueen, Kathleen. 2003.

Community participation and policies of Government of India

In the 1940s, the Bhore Committee espoused the concept of a 'social physician', but this concept was discarded in the Second Five Year Plan. In the Fourth Five Year Plan (1971–75), the expenditure required to strengthen rural health infrastructure was under-funded by Rs 1 billion (Mistry 2003). The Fifth Five Year Plan (1976–80) aimed at opening additional Primary Health

Centres (PHCs), sub centres and rural hospitals. The 'Multi-Purpose Workers Scheme' (MPWs) was introduced, which sought to consolidate all paramedical personnel of various disease control programmes into a single cadre and to integrate different vertical programmes at the village level. In the year 1975, the Srivastava Committee[2] recommended the 'Community Health Worker (CHW) Scheme' for operation at a per 1,000 population level. The CHW was envisaged to be a part time health worker selected by and to work for health issues of her own community. Essentially, she was to be a link between the MPW at the sub centre and the community to provide preventive, promotive and basic curative services (Mistry and Antia 2003).

The Sixth Five Year Plan (1981–85) brought about a further expansion of rural infrastructure, particularly PHCs. As a result of the Alma Ata Declaration, emphasis was placed on an integrated approach to development that included poverty eradication as well as a clear role for the people in determining their health care needs. Furthermore, the report of 'Health for All: An Alternative Strategy 1980' by Indian Council of Social Science Research (ICSSR)/Indian Council of Medical Research (ICMR) emphasised the development of community based integrated health systems inclusive of a graded referral system and nutrition. (ICSSR/ICMR 1980).

The Government of India has adopted certain new policies since the Ninth Five Year Plan (1997–2002) as part of the Family Welfare Programme. Emphasis has been placed on the quality of services; introduction of access, quality and impact indicators; the establishment or reinforcement of financial and managerial decentralisation; and community participation.

Some examples of community participation in India

Jamkhed Rural Health Programme, Maharashtra was the first community based primary health care programme focusing on providing adequate training and support for barely literate women. Dr Arole initiated this unique process in community action that has been nurtured to result as one of the best primary health care models in the world. The programme covers 100,000 people in 70 villages and has documented infant and child mortality reductions in the intervention areas. This project demonstrates the capacity of communities for change and their ability to effectively take on the position of leadership if given the opportunity and support.

The Foundation for Research in Community Health (FRCH) in Maharashtra has focussed on the development of a decentralised, graded, community based and people-centred health care system. FRCH offers unique opportunities for delivering a variety of technologies related to family planning in a safe, cost-effective and humane manner that ensures day-to-day monitoring of users with a high level of technical and counselling skills. FRCH has understood the advantage of a personalised system not only in dispelling mistrust and fear associated with top-down and centralised family planning initiatives, but also in terms of cost-effectiveness.

Society for Education, Action and Research in Community Health (SEARCH) has been working in Gadchiroli, Maharashtra since 1986. Male village health workers (*Arogyadoot*) and Trained Traditional Birth Attendants (TBAs) provide counselling as well as basic care during pregnancy, delivery and post-partum. They also attend to health problems in the region such as pneumonia in children. These interventions have made improvements in maternal and child health that has resulted in the reduction of maternal and neo-natal deaths.

Self Employed Women's Association (SEWA) (Rural) in Gujarat has been focusing on community health programmes aiming to improve maternal and child health since the early 1970s. SEWA's health-related activities are diverse and include primary health care, which is delivered through 60 stationary health centres and mobile health camps; health education and training; capacity building among local SEWA leaders and *dais*; provision of high-quality low-cost drugs through drug shops; occupational and mental health activities; and production and marketing of traditional medicines.

European commission-supported sector investment programme (ECSIP)

ECSIP is an integral part of the Government of India's National Family Welfare Programme. The European Commission (EC) has been supporting SIP since October 1998 with the aim of re-forming the Indian health care system by focusing on primary health care services, including first referral institutions and involving the community. This programme operates at all levels of the system—central, state and district—with emphasis on decentralisation, community involvement in decision making and capacity development of health service providers.

The decentralised management structure set up in the programme such as the Sector Reform Cells at the state level, integrated health and family welfare agencies at the district level and autonomous management bodies at the facility level, is helping to improve the running of primary health centres and referral hospitals. A large number of health functionaries and rural people including women are being trained as part of awareness building. The programme is also supporting improvement of existing national and state government policies and procedures to facilitate delivery of quality health care in the rural and semi-urban areas. Several policy reviews have been undertaken on human resource management and the rational use of infrastructure. The programme is associated with over 40 NGOs and institutions as well as a number of Panchayati Raj Institutions (PRIs). Two important examples of community participation—*Mitanins* and *Sanjeevanis*—implemented in the EC-supported Health and Family Welfare Sector Investment Programme are given in the following section.

The *Mitanin* programme

The rural areas of Chhattisgarh have experienced high prevalence of communicable diseases and low utilisation of public health services. Poor health education, poor access to health services and the prevalent cultural practices have contributed to this. It is only through the strengthening of service delivery and consequently an increase in utilisation rates that this picture could change. To achieve this, the community is encouraged to participate for developing better linkages with health programmes. This is reflected in the Mitanin programme.

The Mitanin programme was announced in November 2001 with the purpose of using community participation for improvement of maternal and child health. A consultative process between the state and the district as well as block levels was adopted for the implementation of the programme. This programme was piloted in 14 community development blocks in May 2002. In January 2003, the programme was expanded to 80 blocks, including the 14 pilot blocks.

Mitanin literally means 'a friend' in the language of Chhattisgarh and surrounding areas. In each hamlet, the community selects a Mitanin, an active woman in the area who is willing and capable to take on the role. This Mitanin acts as a 'change agent' by working as a health activist. To ensure effectiveness of the Mitanin, she is supported at two levels: (a) internally, in the habitation, by the women's health committee, the village health committee and the elected panchayat; and (b) externally, by a cadre of trainers and the government employees who help in building her capacities to perform her functions well. The woman chosen as Mitanin undergoes a 20-day residential training along with 30 days of on-the-job village training.

The significance of the programme lies in the fact that it is not only a means but also as an end in itself. The collateral benefits of training 54,000 Mitanins in 54,000 habitations is to generate awareness in the community, which is by itself a significant achievement. Furthermore, formation of women's habitation committees would be a significant gain not only for the health sector, but for other programmes too.

Role of the Mitanins

As envisaged in the programme, the role of the Mitanins includes:

1. Health education and improving public awareness of health issues among the community members.
2. Improving existing linkages between public health care services.
3. Initiation of collective community level action for health and related development sectors.
4. Identification and provision of immediate relief from common health problems.
5. Organising women for health action and building processes leading to women's empowerment.
6. Sensitising panchayat(s) to build up their understanding and capabilities in local health planning and programme implementation.

Some achievements

Mitanins have been successful in bringing change to remote areas with scant public service facilities and political unrest of the *Naxalites* (extremist groups). Mitanins have started making headway in achieving their arduous goals, as reflected by the following instances:

1. Mitanins have played an important role in expansion of coverage of health services in areas that were under-served. About 530 such hamlets in remote tribal regions have been identified and the gaps between services required and available have been reduced. For example in Manendragarh block of Koriya district, the Mitanins have launched awareness generation as a campaign. They have emerged as strong community leaders and are in dialogue with the state Health Department for the assertion of community needs.
2. Mitanins have helped improve breast feeding practices. As per the cultural norm of some places, the newborn is not breast fed for three days after birth while the mother is not given any water to drink for five days from the time of delivery. The Mitanins' efforts have brought about significant and visible changes in these practices, resulting in immediate post-partum breast-feeding and proper care of the mother.

3. The Mitanins persuade and remind expecting and lactating mothers to avail regular health services like immunisation and antenatal checkups. Thus, they act as a link between the community and service providers such as the Auxillary Nurse Midwife (ANM) and *Aanganwadi* Worker (AWW).

4. In the *Aanganwadi* Centre (AWC) of Village Jhiliberna, Block Pharsabahar, Jaspur district, a Mitanin took initiative to get a new mini AWC opened for poor children to provide benefits from the Integrated Child Development Scheme (ICDS), as the original AWC was located at a distance from their homes.

5. The Mitanins have helped upgrade the Community Health Centre (CHC). In the remote Block of Koylibheda of District Kanker, there were no facilities for Emergency Obstetric Care (EmOC). The Mitanins created awareness among the community members regarding benefits and importance of institutional desliveries, leading to a demand for such facilities. Community mobilisation resulted in upgradation of facilities and availability of round the clock services as well as specialists for EmOC.

6. Mitanins are carrying out 'micro planning' for ante-natal care, care during childbirth and post-partum care. This includes details about mode of transport; appropriate referrals and money for expenses that may be required are pooled in. This planning is done in advance based on the woman's medical history and danger signs.

Apart from the above, there have been some associated activities like formation of Self Help Groups (SHGs). Health related expenditure is one of the primary sources of indebtedness in these areas where organised banking services still remain out of the reach for the majority. This forces them to take loans from the money lenders on exorbitant rate of interests, pushing them further into debt. The formation of such SHGs and regular savings ensure that the women members have a collective amount of money to meet health care needs. This saves them from entering into this vicious cycle of indebtedness. Some women have also come up as entrepreneurs by starting small scale enterprises.

> ### Strong and self employed
> In Pamshala village, a Mitanin borrowed Rs 8,000 at the rate of 2 per cent interest to establish a *dhaba* (a roadside cafe). Apart from returning the money to her group, now she earns a daily profit of Rs 200–300.

Mitanins have brought confidence and equity to existing social relations, not only vis-à-vis health services, but also within their communities. One such example is the 'Anti Liquor Campaign' launched by women under the leadership of Mitanins and SHGs. Mitanins have been elected in the local government PRIs as well. As a result, over 2,000 Mitanins across the state now hold elected offices.[3]

> ### A friend in need, Mitanin indeed
> When Manju became pregnant she was deserted by her husband. She understood her vulnerable condition and the only support for her were Mangini and Rambai, the two Mitanins she knew. Gauging the situation, the two Mitanins raised donations for helping out Manju for the delivery, besides arranging for the necessary medical attention. Simultaneously, they started persuading her husband to accept his wife and child. Manju's delivery was conducted by a trained nurse and the money raised was spent on transport and other necessities. In the meantime, Mangini and Rambai managed to reconcile Manju with her husband. Now Manju lives in her home with her healthy child. The Mitanins provided Manju with critical support in the time of need.

Sanjeevani programme

Haryana is known to have an adverse female-male ratio and low levels of women literacy, making evident the deep gender inequity prevalent in the rigid patriarchal society. In this socio-cultural milieu, a well designed integrated intervention was deemed necessary to raise the social status of women.

The *Sanjeevani* programme was initiated under the Integrated Women Empowerment and Development Programme (IWEDP) in the districts of Mahendragarh and Rewari (Haryana). The ECSIP adopted this programme in three districts of Ambala, Yamunanagar and Karnal in Haryana during mid-2001. The intervention was designed to mobilise women as leaders of social change, generate awareness, initiate social group formation and improve access to health care. A total of 422 women from these districts were identified as Sanjeevanis over a span of two years,[4] and these women were trained for 10 days on issues related to health, particularly maternal and child health, legal issues, community mobilisation and record keeping.

The objectives of the Sanjeevani programme include:

1. development of community leadership qualities, and
2. generating awareness on health issues.

A woman from the community is selected to become a Sanjeevani, by the District Health Officer, State Medical Officer and Medical Officer from the concerned Community Health Centre (CHC). This may include the PRI members wherever possible. The Sanjeevani should be a married woman from the community with at least middle school education.

Roles of Sanjeevanis

The primary roles of the Sanjeevanis include:

1. Generating awareness on better health practices in early childcare and maternal health.
2. Disseminating information regarding mother and child immunisation.
3. Counselling on issues related to family planning, HIV/AIDS, adolescent health.
4. Dispelling myths on health issues (like black magic) that hinder or delay health seeking.

Some achievements

The contribution of Sanjeevanis should be seen in the light of the context they are functioning in. The impact of their inputs may not yet be reflected in health statistics, but they definitely contribute to the overall improvement in health seeking behaviour and practices. Demand for better health facilities and health information are some of the significant outcomes of the Sanjeevani programme. Nonetheless, Sanjeevanis have come out as important community leaders and are looked upon as role models by other women living in a patriarchal social order.

Conclusion

Experiences from the Mitanin and Sanjeevani programmes have brought some challenges to the forefront. These include:

1. Community ownership plays an important role in the sustainability of such endeavours, and therefore, the process for selection of these 'change agents' is critical.
2. Forging strong partnerships between communities and health services so as to meet the increased demand for services with improved supply is crucial for attaining the goal of better health.

Evidence has shown that economic progress alone will not help India achieve the Millennium Development Goals targets. The issues of health and female education will have to be addressed in a holistic manner. Mere increase in government expenditure will not be enough. Civil society and local communities will have to play a larger role in ensuring that the public money is well spent. Child and maternal health are inextricably linked requiring equitable access of stronger quality health systems. The National Rural Health Mission (NRHM) states accessibility to equitable, affordable and effective primary health care with special focus on the poor, women and children, as one of the its prime objectives. Accredited Social Health Activist (ASHA) is adopted as one of the core strategies for effective implementation of the programme. She is envisaged as an interface between the community and the public health systems. In order to ensure that such endeavours are successful, lessons learnt from initiatives such as Mitanins and Sanjeevanis need to be integrated.

Annex 1

MDG Targets	Tenth Plan Target of Government of India	Where is India Today?
Extreme poverty to be halved between 1990 and 2015. Poverty rate in India to be brought down in 2015 to 16 per cent according to international definitions	Incidence of poverty to be brought down to 10 per cent by 2012	The incidence of poverty is around 26 per cent according to Government of India definitions and around 35 per cent according to international definitions
All children to be in primary school by 2015	All children to be in primary school by 2003.	92.14 per cent of children (82.85 per cent for girls) in primary school
Eliminate the difference between male and female literacy by 2007	Halve the difference between male and female literacy by 2007	The literacy rate for men is 74 per cent and for women it is 52 per cent—a difference of 22 per cent
Reduce 1990 mortality rates for infants and children under the age of 5 by two-thirds by 2015 (2015 target for infant deaths: 40 per 1,000)	Reduce infant deaths to 45 per 1,000 births by 2007	Infant deaths: 68 per 1,000 Under-five mortality: 93 per 1,000 births
Reduce deaths due to childbearing (maternal mortality) by three-fourths of 1990 figures by 2015	Reduce deaths due to childbearing to 1 per 1,000 by 2012	Deaths due to childbearing range between 4 to 5.5. per 1,000 births
Halve the proportion of people without safe drinking water (Target: 85 per cent of people get safe drinking water)	All villages to have sustained access to safe drinking water by 2007	84 per cent of rural families and 95 per cent of urban families have access to safe drinking water but not all sources are sustainable

Source: http://southasia.oneworld.net (Accessed in October 2005).

Notes

1. These can be processes and outcomes and all may not be present in a given community participation experience. They are not mutually exclusive.
2. On Medical Education and Support Manpower.
3. 23 *Panch*, 5 *Sarpanch*, 2 *Janpad* members of one block alone started as *Mitanins*.
4. Including refresher trainings.

References

Freedman, Lynn, R. J. Waldman, H. Pinho, M. R. Wirth, A. Mushtaque, R. Chowdhary and A. Rosenfield. 2005. *Who's Got the Power? Transforming Health Systems for Women and Children: Achieving the Millennium Development Goals*. London: Earthscan.

ICSSR and ICMR. 1980. *Health for All–An Alternative Strategy*. Report of a Study Group, ICSSR and ICMR, New Delhi. Submitted to Indian Institute of Education, Pune, August 1980.

Macqueen, Kathleen. 2003. 'Back to the Rough Ground- Community Participation in Ethics Guidelines for HIV Prevention Trials'. Family Health International. Available online at http://www.hptn.org/ResearchEthics/HPTN_Ethics_Guidance.htm (accessed in October 2005).

Macqueen, K. M., Eleanor McLellan, David S. Metzger, Susan Kegeles, Ronald P. Strauss, Roseanne Scotti, Lynn Blanchard and Robert T. Trotter. et al. 2001. 'What is a Community? An Evidence Based Definition for Participatory Public Health', *AJPH*, 91: 1929–38.

Mistry, N. 2003. *Community Based Health Workers—A Review from India*. Mumbai: The Foundation for Research in Community Health.

Outcome Evaluation of the Mitanin Programme. A Critical Assessment of the Nation's Largest Ongoing Community Health Activist Programme based on an objective sample survey of 1219 Mitanins and their work. Chhattisgarh: State Health Resource Centre.

Rivero, David A. 2003. 'Alma-Ata Revisited', *Perspectives in Health Magazine*, 8(2). (http://www.Paho.org/english/dd/pin/Number17_article1_4.htm).

Schuler, S.R., S.M. Hashemi, A. Cullum, M. Hassan. 1996. 'The advent of family planning as a social norm in Bangladesh: women's experiences. Reproductive Health Matters', *International Family Planning Perspectives*, 7: 66–78.

Managing Urban Health through Public-Private Partnership: A Study of Ahmedabad City

16

K.V. Ramani, Dileep Mavalankar,
Amit Patel and Sweta Mehandiratta

Urbanisation

The world's urban population, which accounted for 2 per cent of the population in 1800, increased to nearly 45 per cent of the population by 2000. Today, nearly half the world's population is urban and the urban population is growing by 60 million persons per year, which is about three times the rate of increase in the rural population (Mohan and Dasgupta 2005).

India's urban population of 285 million represents 28 per cent of its total population (Singh et al. 2004). In the 1991–2001 decade, while the Indian population grew at the rate of 2 per cent, urban India grew at 3 per cent, mega cities at 4 per cent and the slum population increased by 5 per cent. This is commonly referred to as the 2-3-4-5 syndrome. The current slum population in India is estimated to be 60 million people, accounting for 21 per cent of the total urban population as per official data. Population projections postulate that slum growth in the future is expected to surpass the capacities of civic authorities to respond to the health and infrastructure needs of this population group. Many recent studies have warned about the possible dangers of increasing prevalence rates of communicable diseases, especially HIV/AIDS in urban areas, if proper attention is not paid to urban planning.

Urban health, India's initiatives

Historically, the focus of the Government of India has been on the development of the rural health system, which has a three-tiered, population-based health delivery structure to cater to the largely rural population. As a result, urban health initiatives of the government have not met existing needs. Urban Family Welfare Centres (UFWCs) have been functioning since the 1960s to provide family welfare services, and Urban Health Posts (UHPs) were established in the 1980s to provide outreach services, primary health care and Reproductive and Child Health (RCH) services particularly in urban slums. Currently, there are about 1,100 UFWCs and 900 Urban Health Posts, to serve an urban population of 285 million, which works out to approximately one UFWC/UHP for an urban population of 140,000. Our rural areas are comparatively much better served, with one Primary Health Centre (PHC) for a population of 30,000.

Urban Health has therefore emerged as a priority in recent Government of India policies and plans. The Ninth Five Year Plan (1997–2002) envisaged the development of a well structured network of urban primary care institutions providing health and family welfare services to the population within 1 km to 3 km of their dwellings (Government of India 1997–2003). In addition to funds provided by the government (municipalities, state and central), externally assisted projects were adopted to achieve this goal. The task of restructuring urban health centres is expected to be completed in the Tenth Five Year Plan (2002–07). A fair amount of financial resources have been allocated by the Ministry of Health and Family Welfare, specifically towards the development of city-wide urban health projects under the Tenth Five Year Plan (Government of India 2002–07). Recognising the urgent need to focus on the health of the vulnerable urban populations, the World Bank supported a Family Welfare urban slums project (Ramana and Lule 2003) to improve health outcomes of an urban poor population of 11.3 million people in four Indian cities: Bangalore, Delhi, Hyderabad and Calcutta. The Environmental Health Project (EHP) of USAID organised a national consultation on 'Improving the Health of the Urban Poor' in June 2003 at Bangalore. This conference provided a platform for dialog amongst policy makers, planners and implementers of urban health programmes. Deliberations and recommendations from the workshop provided valuable guidelines for the urban health component of the RCH II programme, starting in April 2005.

In the Union Budget (2005) of the Government of India, a substantial amount of financial resources has been earmarked for improvement of urban health in seven mega Indian cities: Bombay, Calcutta, Delhi, Chennai, Hyderabad, Bangalore and Ahmedabad (Government of India 2005).

Health care in Ahmedabad city

A status report

Ahmedabad City (also known as Ahmedabad Municipal Corporation, or AMC) is the largest city in Gujarat State and the seventh largest city in India, with a population of 3.5 million spread across 192 sq km. The population growth in Ahmedabad over the last five decades is given in Table 16.1.

Table 16.1 Population growth in Ahmedabad

Census year	Population	Decadal growth rate
1951	837,163	41.59 %
1961	1,149,918	37.36 %
1971	1,586,544	37.88 %
1981	2,059,725	29.90 %
1991	2,876,710	20.80 %
2001	3,515,361	22.20 %

Source: Ahmedabad Municipal Corporation 2002a.

The city of Ahmedabad has nearly 7 million dwelling units, of which almost 50 per cent are situated in 2,500 slums (and chawls), housing approximately 1.5 million people. This is the most vulnerable group of the society and needs special attention.

The civic affairs of the city are governed by the Ahmedabad Municipal Corporation (AMC). Administratively, the AMC is divided into 43 Municipal Election Wards across five zones, with each ward having an average population of 80,000 people. These 43 wards elect a total of 129 councillors, who in turn elect a Mayor. The Mayor is chairman of the AMC Board, which makes all policy decisions, and he or she is assisted by a Deputy Mayor, three statutory committees and 13 sub committees. The Municipal Commissioner, who is a civil servant from the Indian Administrative Service, is responsible for executing all decisions taken by the AMC Board. He or she is assisted by nine Deputy Municipal Commissioners: five Deputy Municipal Commissioners for the five zones (Central, East, West, North and South) and one Deputy Municipal Commissioner each for Engineering, Security, Administration and Finance. One of the nine zonal deputy municipal commissioners is given the additional charge of running Health Department. The organisational chart of the Health Department at AMC is shown in Exhibit 1.

The AMC attaches considerable significance to health care, allocates 10–12 per cent of its annual budget to the health sector and subsidises the cost of health care by offering services through its network of 70 centres, composed of family welfare centres, dispensaries, maternity homes and general hospitals (Ahmedabad Municipal Corporation 2002b). The state government of Gujarat has a large Civil hospital, with more than 2,000 beds, in Ahmedabad city. The Employee State Insurance (ESI) Corporation of the Government of India administers its scheme through 50 ESI dispensaries and 2 ESI hospitals in Ahmedabad.

A GIS map showing the locations of public health care facilities in Ahmedabad reveals some very interesting observations. There are wide variations in the quality of health care services in various parts of the city. Most health facilities are confined to the original 100 sq km area of Ahmedabad city, while the additional area of 92 sq km added to the city limits in 1986 is still very poorly served. Seven out of 43 wards in AMC have no public health facility at all, not even a Family Welfare Centre (see Exhibit 2). It is also apparent that only 1.8 million of the total population of 3.5 million is served by the existing 36 family welfare centres. Certain important indicators of the health status of Ahmedabad city are given in Table 16.2.

Exhibit 1

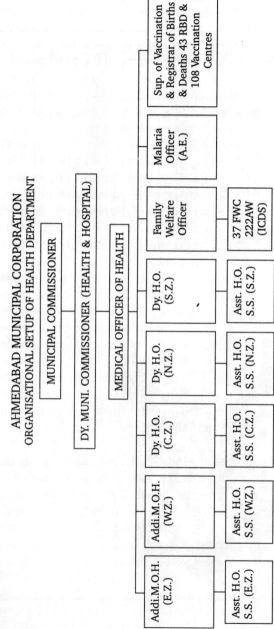

AHMEDABAD MUNICIPAL CORPORATION
ORGANISATIONAL SETUP OF HEALTH DEPARTMENT

MUNICIPAL COMMISSIONER

DY. MUNI. COMMISSIONER (HEALTH & HOSPITAL)

MEDICAL OFFICER OF HEALTH

| Addi.M.O.H. (E.Z.) | Addi.M.O.H. (W.Z.) | Dy. H.O. (C.Z.) | Dy. H.O. (N.Z.) | Dy. H.O. (S.Z.) | Family Welfare Officer | Malaria Officer (A.E.) | Sup. of Vaccination & Registrar of Births & Deaths 43 RBD & 108 Vaccination Centres |

| Asst. H.O. S.S. (E.Z.) | Asst. H.O. S.S. (W.Z.) | Asst. H.O. S.S. (C.Z.) | Asst. H.O. S.S. (N.Z.) | Asst. H.O. S.S. (S.Z.) | 37 FWC 222AW (ICDS) |

Budget: Health Preventive Sanitation Services   77 Crores
Hospitals-Curative Services   84 Crores
Total Budget   161 Crores

ABBREVIATIONS:
Addi. M.O.H. = Additional Medical Officer of Health
Dy. H.O.   = Deputy Health Officer
Asst. H.O. = Assistant Health Officer
C.Z. = Central Zone, W.Z. = West Zone, E.Z. = East Zone, N.Z. = North Zone, S.Z. = South Zone

Exhibit 2

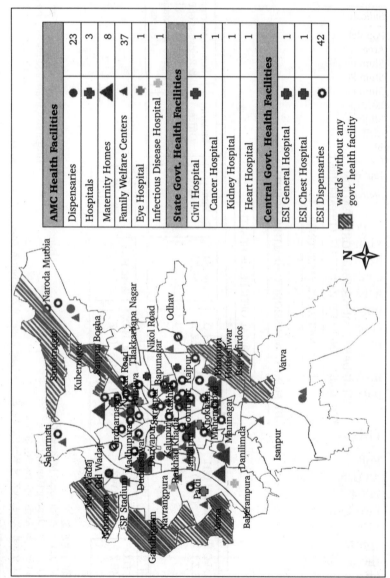

AMC Health Facilities		
Dispensaries	●	23
Hospitals	✚	3
Maternity Homes	◀	8
Family Welfare Centers	▲	37
Eye Hospital	✚	1
Infectious Disease Hospital	✚	1
State Govt. Health Facilities		
Civil Hospital	✚	1
Cancer Hospital		1
Kidney Hospital		1
Heart Hospital		1
Central Govt. Health Facilities		
ESI General Hospital	✚	1
ESI Chest Hospital	✚	1
ESI Dispensaries	○	42

wards without any govt. health facility

Table 16.2   Certain indicators of health status

Indicators	Value
Population	3.5 million
Area	192 sq km
Slum Population	1.5 million
Slum Pockets	2432
Slum Families	3.30,000
IMR (per 1000 live births)	28.6 (2001)
MMR (per 100,000 live births)	130 (2001)
CDR	7.50 (2001)
BR	23.40 (2001)
CPR	56.70 (2001)
Immunisation	80 per cent

Source: Ahmedabad Municipal Corporation 2002b.

Private health care facilities in Ahmedabad are growing rapidly. Ahmedabad city has a large network of more than 3,500 private health care facilities, including a large number of outpatient clinics and small nursing homes. However, it is not possible to get a list of private health facilities, as the private sector in health is not regulated, and there is no mandatory requirement for any clinic/small nursing home in the private sector to be formally registered with the Department of Health.

The large network of public and private sector health facilities in Ahmedabad offers several opportunities for public-private participation to improve the delivery of health services.

Urban health centres

Following the Government of India guidelines, the AMC set up 43 Urban Health Centres (UHCs), one for each ward, on April 2, 2004. This was achieved by upgrading the existing Family Welfare Centres and bringing the UHCs under the administration of an autonomous body, the urban RCH Society. Each UHC is contracted out to a Non-governmental Organisation (NGO), called the mother NGO, for service delivery, which in turn is assisted by a field NGO providing community outreach services.

The AMC attaches one Medical Officer, one Health Visitor, one lab technician and a few Multi Purpose Workers (at the rate of one

Multi Purpose Worker per 20,000 population) to each of these mother NGOs for delivery of health services (see Figure 16.1). Besides these full time employees, one gynecologist and one paediatrician from AMC visit each UHC for a few hours every day. AMC also provides some administrative staff, funds for medicines and drugs, as well as a monthly rent of up to Rs 10,000 to the mother NGOs managing the UHCs.

Figure 16.1   Medical and paramedical staff resources for urban health centre

Urban Health Centre (UHC) for a sample ward

Medical Officer	(AMC)	
Auxiliary Nurse Midwife	(AMC)	UHC Management
Multi Purpose Worker (1 per 10,000 Pop.)	(AMC)	(Mother NGO)
Community Health Worker (Link Worker) (1 Per 2000 Pop.)	(NGO)	

Source: Ahmedabad Municipal Corporation 2002a.

Multi Purpose Workers (MPWs), are trained health workers who provide preliminary medical care (vaccination, injections etc.) to needy patients identified and reported by the link workers. They accompany link workers in turn (one MPW for three to four Link Workers), spend four days in the field that includes one day per week on immunisation camps, and are also responsible for maintaining a large number of registers (data on their community services) and generating reports. Link workers, who are from the slum community in the same ward, visit the slums daily to assess community needs and promote health awareness and prevention measures. Their work involves facilitating IEC, awareness, and motivation campaigns; serving as a link between their community and the UHC-MPW for RCH and primary health services; collecting blood smear of fever cases; and providing treatment (DOT) to TB patients, etc.

The work of UHCs will be supervised by the zonal administration through a Deputy Municipal Commissioner and Deputy

Health Officers in each zone. A Medical Officer of Health (MOH) will have the overall responsibility for the entire range of health services.

Urban health centre for Vasna ward

The existing UHC

It can be seen from Exhibit 2 that Vasna ward has no government health facility. Vasna, with its population of 1 lakh people, 40 per cent of whom live in slums, has its UHC located in Paldi, the adjacent ward.

Vasna UHC is managed by an NGO, the Akhand Jyot Foundation, which has been in charge of a Family Welfare Centre in Vasna since 1966. The existing Family Welfare (FW) centre was upgraded into a UHC in June 2004, supplemented by some additional resources from the RCH Society. Link workers for the Vasna UHC are provided by SAATH, an NGO that has been very active in the Vasna ward for a number of years.

The quality of health services to the poor of Vasna is very unsatisfactory. Availability of UHC services to Vasna population is very bad, as its UHC is located in the adjacent ward. The existing location of the Vasna UHC in Paldi ward is about 1.5 km away for 15 per cent of the Vasna slum population and is 3.2 km away for 70 per cent of the slum population. Hence, access to UHC services is also inadequate for the Vasna slum population. The slum population in Vasna therefore depends on private health care providers whose charges range from Rs 50 to Rs 100 for consultation and some medication. For investigation services (lab and radiology), they are referred to private facilities, which have high user charges. The above remarks on availability, access, and affordability indicate inequity in health services for the slum population of Vasna.

Proposed UHC: Public-private partnership

As Vasna ward is very poorly served by government health facilities, it would be worthwhile to explore a public-private partnership to better serve the Vasna population.

As a first step, we developed a GIS map of Vasna ward that charted all the private health facilities. We then conducted a health facility survey to understand the range and quality of services offered by these private providers. We also held extensive discussions with all stakeholders involved: AMC, private health care providers, elected representatives, and the slum population, in order to assess the health care needs of the Vasna community. We identified the Community Oncology Centre (COC) managed by the Gujarat Cancer Society as an ideal facility to locate the Vasna UHC. It can be seen from Exhibit 3 that almost 70 per cent of the Vasna slum population can be covered within a 1 km

Exhibit 3   Service level at proposed location at Community Oncology Centre

Service Level for Vasna UHC at COC

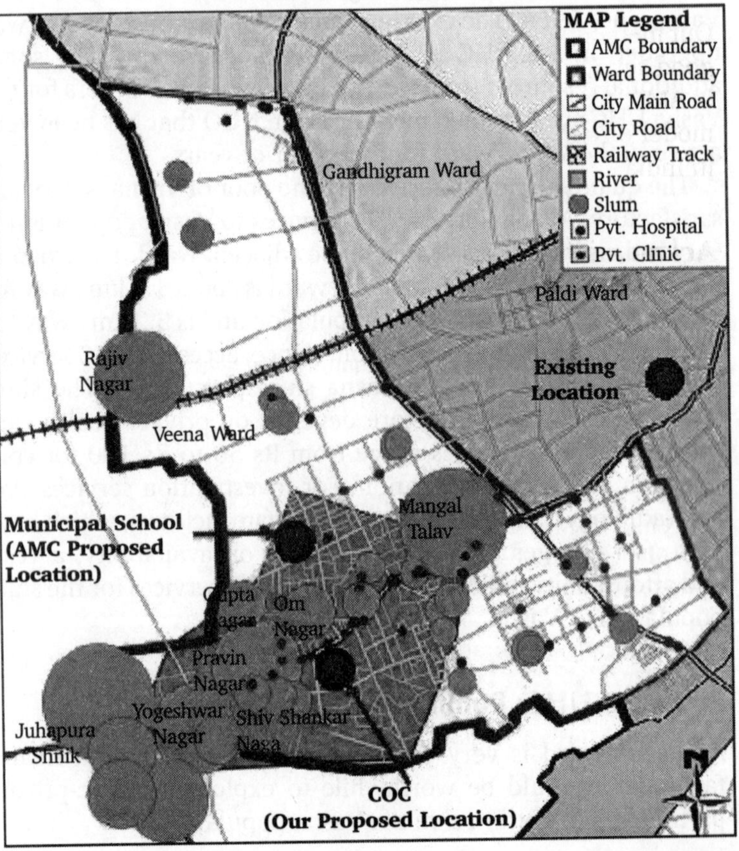

distance from the COC. Additionally, the COC also has excellent laboratory and radiology facilities, a community hall for health promotional activities, is easily accessible by road and has a good reputation in the area.

We have now established a public-private partnership between the Ahmedabad Municipal Corporation and the Gujarat Cancer Society (GCS), whereby the GCS will build an UHC and handover its operations to the AMC. The existing contract between AMC, Akhand Jyot Foundation (mother NGO) and SAATH Field NGO) has been suitably modified for Vasna UHC services to be offered from the new UHC located in GCS compound, Vasna.

Conclusion

Our methodology of relying on GIS to identify ideal locations and good service providers is now being extended to another ward in AMC. Based on our experience, we hope to develop a working model of public-private partnership in managing urban health in India.

Acknowledgement

We would like to thank Ahmedabad Municipal Corporation and SAATH for their excellent assistance in carrying out this study. We would also like to acknowledge UNFPA for funding this research project.

References

Ahmedabad Municipal Corporation. 2002a. *Urban Reproductive and Child Health Care Project in the city of Ahmedabad*. Ahmedabad: Ahmedabad Municipal Corporation.

———. 2002b. *Statistical Outline of Ahmedabad City 2000–2001*, Ahmedabad: Planning and Statistics Department, Ahmedabad Municipal Corporation.

Ninth Five Year Plan 1997–03; Government of India.

Ramana GNV and Elizabeth Lule. 2003. 'Improving health outcomes among urban poor-The challenges and opportunities: Lessons from India Family Welfare Urban Slums project', paper presented at the Urban Research Symposium entitled Urban Development for Economic Growth and Poverty Reduction by World Bank,

Washington DC, 15–17 December 2003. Available online at http://www.worldbank.org/urban/symposium2003/docs/papers/ramana.pdf

Rakesh Mohan and Shubhagato Dasgupta. 2005. 'The 21st century: Asia Becomes Urban', in *Economic and Political Weekly*, Vol. XL(3): 213–223.

Singh Anju Dadhwal, Shivani Taneja and Sidharth Agarwal. 2004. *Technical Assistance to the Government of India for Urban Health Planning and National Guidelines,* Activity report 135, EHP, Environmental Health Project, USAID (Unpublished document).

Tenth Five Year Plan 2002–07; Government of India.

Union Budget. 2005, Government of India.

Standards of Medical Care: Is India Ready?

17

MICHAEL FRIEDMAN

Introduction

In spite of the rapidly increasing prevalence of HIV/AIDS, India is still ill-prepared to tackle the threat of this disease. Therefore, the main issue lies in making apparent the necessity of dealing with this epidemic. In the US, which has less than a million people affected with HIV/AIDS, there are thousands of experts working on the disease. However, in India, with more than 5 million HIV/AIDS victims, there is inadequate capacity for management of the ailment. Although there is extensive media coverage, political commitment is lacking. Improvement is needed in; the standardisation of common medical practices, the accreditation processes of health care delivery, management skills, systems development and in establishing accountability, as it is missing in the current system. Developing innovative methods for scaling-up quality standards is one way to improve health conditions. This chapter focuses on the need to improve the quality of medical care in India.

Centers for Disease Control and Prevention (CDC)

The Centers for Disease Control and Prevention (CDC) is the US government agency responsible for ensuring the health of its citizens. Although 95 per cent of its work is focussed within US borders, CDC has a long history of providing technical assistance to other countries in relation to various public health issues such as Smallpox, Polio, TB, SARS, Avian Flu and HIV. Currently, its main programmatic activity in India and throughout the world is in providing assistance for implementation of effective HIV prevention and care activities. This programme is called CDC's Global AIDS Programme (GAP). As a part of its mission in India, CDC believes that a broader look at both the functionality and quality of the entire health system is necessary in order to develop quality and sustainable HIV care programmes. Thus, HIV has been an example of the potential role for standards of care and accreditation systems within India. With the growing privatisation of health care services, it is now time to develop and field-test innovative approaches to the 'accountability question'.

The prime principle is to develop screening at the grassroots level, as small towns are the main focus group and are more susceptible to HIV. As far as quality of service is concerned, efficient use of existing infrastructure and strict monitoring and evaluations are required.

Standards of HIV care in India

This chapter outlines the core elements of quality HIV care in Indian medical institutions (clinics, nursing homes, hospitals). This is meant for all medical practitioners who care for persons living with HIV/AIDS (PLHAs), whether they consider themselves to be local/regional experts in HIV/AIDS or are just beginning to address this disease in their medical practice.

Standards of care are generally developed in order to set a 'minimum' standard of care for a particular disease/condition. These standards are usually compiled from the best available scientific evidence for treating each condition, from more holistic understandings of that disease and from general medical practice standards in that country. Unlike medical guidelines, standards of care are not intended to describe in detail the diagnosis, treatment and care of every aspect of the disease. Instead, they are used to assist medical practitioners and administrators to set priorities for care, evaluate their own care systems and gain an understanding of the most essential aspects of care.

The HIV care standards for India are intended to be similar to other standard of care documents. They are specifically designed for the modern Indian health care system, that is, for the private 'for-profit' sector, NGO 'non-profit' sector and government sector. Some may find these basic standards of care easier to implement in large urban hospitals versus in understaffed rural dispensaries. Regardless, these HIV standards of care should help to understand the most important aspects of caring for PLHAs; set priorities for establishing or expanding HIV care practices; maximise the efficiency and time of medical staff in addressing HIV/AIDS; establish a system for evaluating and/or monitoring HIV care practices in a particular clinic/hospital on a larger scale; and to promote certain HIV/AIDS medical care institutions that meet standards.

In addition, consumer rights organisations, advocacy groups, networks of positive persons, hospital administrators and civic leaders can use this document to promote quality HIV care that is standardised and measurable. PLHAs and their families will have realistic expectations of their medical care providers, and in turn, medical care providers will be issued clear expectations from HIV training programmes and from the leaders of India's health care systems.

Accreditation

Accreditation is the process of setting minimally acceptable standards for a specified field of service (that is, medical care) and then periodically evaluating the providers of that service in a pre-set, transparent and structured way to determine if both the service and its delivery meet those standards.

Health care accreditation should objectively measure the most meaningful aspects of patient care, including, but not limited to, important measures of health outcomes that reflect the quality of services provided. It may also measure administrative and structural processes such as Total Quality Improvement (TQI) systems and patient flow. The Indian health care system requires accreditation, as it increases transparency and accountability, rewards quality medical practice, sets needed standards and teaches continuous quality improvement concepts. Organisation and regulation of the private health care sector empowers patients (consumers of health care) by providing them with valuable information for action, which leads to better medical practice, an important requirement of accreditation.

Standards of care

A critical question arises: 'How will health care providers and institutions follow standards of care?' The answer is that multiple creative strategies are necessary to get any standard of care document to be followed and practised. There are several ways to influence (and ultimately improve) the behaviours of medical practitioners and the health care system in general. A common method is to improve the knowledge of medical professionals regarding the science of a particular disease or health issue. This is the rational for conducting all kinds of classroom-based trainings, seminars, conferences and workshops and is also the basis for medical journals and textbooks. Knowledge is a key component of providing quality medical care, but knowledge alone is not enough, as it does not necessarily equal behaviour change. While creating a microenvironment (in hospitals or clinics) where high quality medical care is easier to practise, this may also influence the health care system. This includes few examples as:

1. setting up continuous quality improvement mechanisms (also called Total Quality Management [TQM]),
2. hiring support staff to assist doctors in areas where a physician's skills or time is limited (that is, for nutritional support, counselling, etc.) and a clinic manager with hospital administration skills,
3. creating simple flow sheets or assessment forms for evaluating and tracking patients, and
4. using visual aids to remind physicians to use specific care-related practices.

This 'system' approach for changing a physician's behaviour can be extremely effective if the 'system' is improved. However, resources are needed to do the work properly, and if senior management does not feel that there is much 'return on investment,' this may not happen.

However, another option for quality improvement could be implementation of penalties for poor quality medical practices. This requires agreement on what determines a good or bad quality medical practice, a system for identifying poor practices, and a way to punish those whose practise is of poor quality. The best example is the medico-legal system, where poor practices are dealt with via lawsuits. Other examples include revoking medical licenses or hospital privileges and termination from services, which are all relatively uncommon and are reserved for only the most outlandishly poor medical practices. Nevertheless, incentives for good quality medical services are the best way to influence the system. The best example, which is currently in practise, is the free market health sector economy, where consumers can choose doctors and hospitals that ideally provide better care services. However, market decisions on health care are more often based upon cost, convenience, culture and incorrect assumptions about quality of care than on well-thought out and standardised indicators of quality medical care. If this is to work optimally, this strategy needs to change. Some progress has been made in India with the adoption of advanced medical degrees (post-graduate degree holders generally are more in demand and can charge more as compared to MBBS doctors) and International Organization of Standardisation (ISO 9000) certification of hospitals.

Creating an accreditation system based on formulated standards of care can be an effective tool for creating good physicians and hospitals, because if it works well, it can incorporate all of the above strategies into one specific programme. Standards of care help to increase knowledge by making learning more focussed and efficient. Standards can also create change in clinics or in hospital-level systems by constructing criterion that must be achieved. Accreditation builds a system for all this and more importantly, an incentive, which is necessary if consumers and the medical community in general are to value this. Finally, it is a system that empowers health care consumers to make better decisions about medical care services, which in turn drives the health care system to improve its quality of practices.

There are a few action steps for implementation of an accreditation system based on standards of care. Concise, well-articulated documents that describe standards of care that are reality-based and have broad buy-in by leaders of Indian clinical care must be drafted, just as it is necessary to obtain an official 'stamp of approval' for the standard of care by key organisations. A mechanism needs to be created for dissemination of these standards to a wide circle of physicians and hospitals. The dissemination process should focus on training medical providers on details of the standards as well as on practical ways to reach these standards through realistic, easily implemented system changes. By using this as a training opportunity, accreditation can be explained to medical providers.

The standards must be simplified while a mechanism is created to promote these care standards to consumers of health care who have that specific medical condition. Trainings or classes on understanding these standards, and also on how to determine if a doctor is practicing them, need to be developed in a creative way (that is, utilisation of audio-visual materials, simple pamphlets or posters listing the standards, etc.). A system should be formulated for assessing how well medical sites/providers follow standards, and this monitoring/assessment system needs to be objective, consistent and not too laborious. It also needs to be field tested in multiple sites. A system of assessment tools should be developed for accreditation on standards of care, and subsequently, guidelines need to be set on minimum qualifications, frequency of re-accreditation, etc. A system for training assessors and payment scales for their prompt assessment of potential accreditation sites needs to be formed. Last, a formal process of applying for accreditation must be produced, with discussion on whether fees should be charged.

An assessment of the benefits of accreditation must be established both in terms of financial as well as non-financial incentives (that is, better peer or community recognition, staff satisfaction for being part of an innovative process etc.). The first step is assessment of other accreditation systems in India

(ISO 9000 for example), followed by documentation of benefits and disadvantages of going through the newly established care accreditation process. Marketing of the accreditation to both medical providers (including hospital administrators) and consumers is necessary so that motivation for accreditation is increased.

In the international meeting on accreditation, there were examples from South Africa but none from India. A large, undisciplined private sector in India is not sufficient, as involvement of the private sector is equally important. There are a few good examples of accreditation systems throughout the world, which include lab accreditation (Clinical Laboratory Improvement Amendments (CLIA), National Accreditation Board for Laboratories (NABL), American Board of Pathology), hospital accreditation (Joint Commission on Accreditation of Healthcare Organisations [JCAHO]), organizational accreditation (ISO 9000+), drug and pharmaceutical accreditation (Food and Drugs Administration (FDA)), World Health Organization (WHO), medical college accreditation (Medical Council of India (MCI)) and disease-specific accreditations such as standards of care available for diabetes, asthma, emergency trauma care (trauma center levels) and TB (the Revised National TB Control Programme [RNTCP] has standards and a site assessment process established but no formal accreditation practice).

Need for initiation of accreditation in HIV care

Anti-Retroviral Therapy (ART) roll-out is a good opportunity for establishing government-led accreditation systems for all ART delivery sites. India, with 5 million HIV positive people, must learn from systems begun in South Africa, Kenya, Thailand and Uganda, as these systems demonstrate potential ways to get large, undisciplined private sectors involved in quality HIV care.

Accreditation in HIV care: Key issues to resolve

There are various key issues for accreditation of HIV care that must be addressed and subsequently resolved. It is important to determine which model of HIV care is best: the government regulatory model or the voluntary 'corporate' model, with the answer depending on whomever is ready to take the lead on HIV care (though both models can be tested in India). Another issue is that of human capacity limits: when we talk of accreditation, the question arises as to whether India has enough health accreditation experts and high quality site assessors to support a transparent and fair process. It is difficult to know whether the market demand for HIV or 'infectious disease' health care services is similar to that for other disease like diabetes or heart disease. Again, analysis is required to determine the feasibility of accreditation in rural India, where market competition with the government sector is less.

In a study in rural Andhra Pradesh, the organisation found that the system with the best reach is that of the government. The government collaborates with both the CDC and PHC's to provide health services that can better reach un-served populations. Existing PHC staff are already overburdened, and the only solution is to build special HIV services by adding staff and equipment. Nurses are working advocates at the field level, establishing a good political commitment and grassroots reach, and outreach workers also are employed to work with nurses. Another example is Tamil Nadu, where Self Help Group (SHG) women act as outreach workers who raise awareness, and as awareness fails in isolation, the programme also incorporates sexuality, sexual relations, HIV awareness, HIV stigma and community mobilisation. The approach was pilot tested and shown to be successful and there are currently 1,700,000 SHGs in Tamil Nadu that will be trained in programme over the next six months in collaboration with the government.

TB Centre (Madras): It is the biggest HIV centre in the world, and people's awareness is raised here in the natural environment. Other interventions that occur here include a 1 year training on HIV for medical doctors for development of experts in the field. The plan here is to develop a model that can be replicated with future further progression.

In this perspective, the question arises about how to take ideas and actively implement them. On the medical system side, it is important to understand the role of classroom learning—in other countries, unlike in India, doctors need to renew their license.

Some trainings exist that have continuous impact, but in today's scenario, there is a need to have more active learning through use of peer education. TQI is another concern, as regulations and accountability make a difference in inspection of health systems. Other issues involve group dynamics or peer pressure, financial incentives, environmental changes, legal pressures for accountability and Outpatient Department (OPD) drug availability.

Use of standards of care for conditions beside HIV

In fact, standards of care have been mostly used for chronic disease conditions such as diabetes, asthma, heart disease and emergency trauma care. However, the 'standard of care' and accreditation concept has also been widely used and accepted in laboratory medicine, and many accreditation bodies (CLIA, American Board of Pathology, etc.) have existed for years. Another prominent example of the power of accreditation is JCAHO, which accredits entire hospitals, clinics and sometimes just individual departments within a medical care center. All hospitals providing medical care in the United States are required by US law to receive JCAHO approval every few years. JCAHO accreditation is now being sought by large international health care centers such as Apollo hospitals (Delhi and Chennai). However, current efforts at accreditation are limited to their laboratories.

In developing countries, the closest example of a successful standard of care and accreditation system might be the RNTCP. Simple, practical standards for TB diagnosis and care have been established and promoted along with an intensive monitoring system. Thus, RNTCP acts as kind of an informal accreditation body for each Directly Observed Treatment Short Course (DOTS) treatment center and microbiology-testing center. However, there has been little attention paid to developing 'market incentives' for private physicians and hospitals to adopt the RNTCP guidelines, resulting in limited acceptance of the programme in the private health care sector to date. This chapter can be concluded with the lines of Mager, whose writing can provide insight on the present situation: 'If you are not certain of where you are going...you may very well end up somewhere else (and not even know it)'.

Challenges and Approaches towards the Control of Chronic Diseases in a Developing Country with Cancer as a Model

18

A. NANDAKUMAR

Introduction

With the control of communicable diseases and recent changes in lifestyle, non-communicable diseases are emerging as a major public health concern. The incidence of cancer, diabetes, cardiovascular disease, stroke and other neurological diseases are expected to rise in the coming decades. The rising burden of chronic disease is estimated to account for 53 per cent of all deaths and 44 per cent of Disability Adjusted Life Years (DALY) lost in the year 2005 (Reddy et al. 2005). Therefore, there is an urgent need to develop policies and strategies to establish control over chronic diseases in a systematic way.

The term 'control' encompasses a variety of connotations, ranging from reduction of the burden of disease to appropriate management of disease. Another aspect entails defining appropriate standards of treatment, namely for providing post-diagnosis treatment and monitoring post-treatment quality of life. A question often arises, however, about the availability of sufficient databases with which to measure the level of control, achieved. Facts and figures about a disease and its outcome are fundamental for planning, designing, monitoring and eva-luating any health care-directed activity. In addition, they are necessary for assessing costs and setting priorities. Developing countries, including India, do not have a ready and valid national disease database for research, assessing clinical management or monitoring public health control measures. Some reasons for not having accurate databases for estimating the burden of disease involve unsystematic documentation of medical records as discharge summaries, methods of referral and follow-up, the system of registration and certification of the cause of death.

The initial steps for disease control, begin with development of a system that will provide disease related information and a well laid out overall disease control plan with local practical models. The advent of Information Technology (IT) has an impact in several fields. In a developing country like India, its reach in the health sector is visible in components of diagnostic reports and as a part of patient management tools, especially in the private sector. Advances in electronic IT and principles of modern management need to be harnessed. This will help to provide, complete, high quality and valid data. Additionally, consolidation of existing information will generate an instrument for disease control and research that will influence health care delivery and foster health informatics.

Cancer control

In our country, there are two major lacunae in the control of disease: lack of systematic study and lack of measurable parameters on the burden of disease. Action, measures, strategies and priorities should be based on scientific evidence that combines knowledge from recent advances in medicine, application of research results, epidemiological findings, statistical data and periodic situational analyses and projections. Necessary material must be developed in order to promote awareness and the need for 'control'.

While considering the example of Cancer, Doctors Greenwald and Cullen wrote in 1985: 'Cancer Control is the reduction of cancer incidence, morbidity and mortality through an orderly sequence from research on intervention and their impact on defined populations to the broad systematic application of the research results' (Greenwald and Cullen 1985).

There is a need to minimise incidence and mortality from cancer while placing emphasis on people's quality of life, the efficiency of cancer services and developing measurable indicators. Currently, there is token documentation of hospital records on cancer. The baseline parameters required for monitoring performance of control programmes are: the magnitude and patterns of disease; types of risk factors that include age, sex and state/district-wide geographic variations; the level of disease at diagnosis; and trends in incidence, mortality and survival or cure rate.

To understand any disease, particularly cancer, an idea of the magnitude of the problem is essential. Knowing variation in patterns across geographic areas and populations helps in better comprehension of the disease. Changes in magnitude and patterns over time also contribute to its perception. Correlation of these parameters with habits and lifestyle of the population provide clues to causes of disease. This in essence is cancer registration and epidemiology. Cancer registration is a means to a purpose and not a purpose in itself. It is the forerunner of studies in descriptive epidemiology of cancer, which in turn generate specific scientific hypotheses. Studying the magnitude and patterns of cancer would be the first step in determining clues to the cause of cancer and having a baseline to plan and assess control measures. Epidemiologic studies based on these help in knowing what is happening and what can be done about it. Cancer registries provide the needed information to undertake such investigations.

Registration is therefore the rational approach to any disease control programme. As defined, cancer registration involves continuing and systematic data collection on the occurrence and characteristics of reportable neoplasms (MacLennan et al. 1978).

1. *Continuing is the* main feature that distinguishes cancer registration from a cancer survey, which is for a limited period of time.
2. *Systematic data collection* implies complete coverage of the various sources of cancer cases in a given population.

There are different types of Cancer Registries, namely population based, hospital based and those for special purposes such as exposure, site, paediatrics or specific morphologies (mesothelioma). Dr Jussawala of the Indian Cancer Society started the first cancer registration programme in India during 1964, in Bombay. The National Cancer Registry Programme (NCRP) of the Indian Council of Medical Research (ICMR) began in 1981. The programme has laid a strong foundation over the years for the construction of a database for cancer disease. Setting up and identifying Regional Cancer Centres across the country has contributed enormously to the dissemination of information on cancer and improved opportunities for organised treatment, and the system demonstrates a vast potential for research and control of cancer. The advent of electronic IT and its use in evolving an Atlas of cancer in India gives a new dimension to disease data collation.

As of now in India we have 21 population based and five hospital based cancer registries in India and this is depicted in Map 18.1. The entire registry programme of the country is coordinated and directed by the NCRP office located in Bangalore.

Geographic trends in cancer in India

Data on cancer collected from male populations in the six older population based cancer registries (operating from the years 1982 or 1988), reveal that stomach cancer was the leading site in Bangalore and Chennai, whereas hypopharynx, tongue and lung cancer were the leading sites in Barshi, Bhopal, Mumbai and Delhi respectively. In 2001, stomach cancer remained the leading site in Bangalore and Chennai, oesophagus cancer at Barshi and lung cancer in Bhopal while remaining high in Delhi and Mumbai. When looking at the leading sites of cancer among women in the above six registries, it is observed that cancer of the cervix was high in Bangalore, Bhopal and Chennai during the year 1982 or 1988. During 2001, in Barshi, the incidence of cervix cancer decreased. It was surpassed by breast cancer in other places. The proportion of cervical and breast cancer remained high at all points of time in all registries.

Trends in the age-adjusted incidence rate (AAR) of cancer show a rise in the incidence of gallbladder cancer in Delhi. Similarly, the rate of incidence of breast and ovarian cancer increased

Map 18.1 **Shows locations of various population based and hospital based registries in India**

NATIONAL CANCER REGISTRY PROGRAMME

(*Indian Council of Medical Research*)

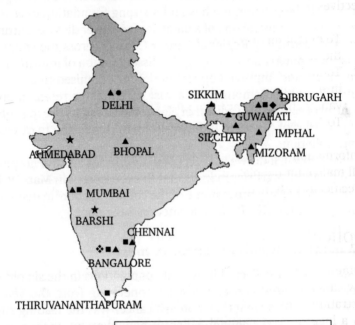

- ● ICMR HEADQUARTERS
- ❖ NCRP COORDINATING UNIT
- ▲ POPULATION BASED REGISTRY
- ★ POPULATION BASED RURAL REGISTRY
- ■ HOSPITAL BASED REGISTRY
- ◆ MONITORING UNIT OF NERCR

steadily in Delhi and Mumbai. A decline was observed in the incidence of cervical cancer through the years. An increasing trend in cancer of the prostate is also seen cancers related to the brain and nervous system, such as Non-Hodgkin's Lymphoma, show an increase over time. Comparison of AAR between North Eastern PBCRs (Population Based Cancer Registry) with PBCRs under NCRP (All Sites (ICD-10: C00-C96)-Male and Female both) shows high incidence of all types of cancer in the north-eastern districts as compared to rest of India. The reporting of stomach and lung cancer was very high (approximately 45 per cent) in Aizwal District of Mizoram when compared with other districts in India.

The NCRP has developed an Atlas of cancer in India (Nandakumar et al. 2005) with the support of the WHO. The objectives of the Atlas are:

1. To obtain an overview of the cancers in different parts of the country,
2. To identify similarities and differences in cancer patterns in a relatively cost effective way while using recent advances in electronic/computer IT, and
3. To calculate estimates of cancer incidence wherever feasible.

Information on patient identification and diagnostic details of all malignant neoplasms is entered in a prescribed format on a specifically designed website.

Application of Information Technology (IT)

In January 2002, two websites, www.canceratlasindia.org and www.cancermapindia.org, were developed to allow online registration of new centres. Collaborating centres are provided with a login ID and password regarding online data entry on core forms for onward transmission. A few basic checks on data entry are also provided. The following two maps give information regarding the distribution of collaborating centres, registered centres and centres contacted but not responded, along with the participating centres. Presently, there are 116 collaborating centres in the network (Maps 18.2 and 18.3).

Data received

The data on 217,174 cases was received through these centres (approximately 1,000–1,200 cases per week) between 1st January 2001 and 31st December 2002. Data has also been received in the shape of floppy disk and hard copies of completed forms.

Map 18.2   Map showing distribution of collaborating centres, registered centres and centres contacted but not responded

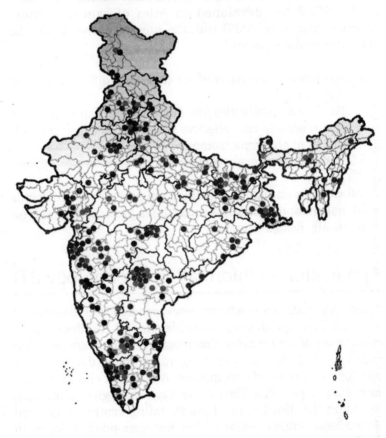

International comparison of AAR with PBCRs under NCRP reveals that prevalence of mouth cancer in men is highest in Bhopal as compared to other parts of the world. However, inter-district comparison of (Minimum Incidence Rates) MAAR with PBCRs under NCRP shows that Wardha District of Maharashtra bears the highest Incidence of mouth cancer, at 14 per 100,000, whereas Bhopal is sixth with an incidence of 9/100,000. Incidence of gallbladder cancer among women in Delhi is the highest, not only in India, but throughout the world. Lung cancer in women is

Map 18.3   Map showing participating centres represented by dots (•)

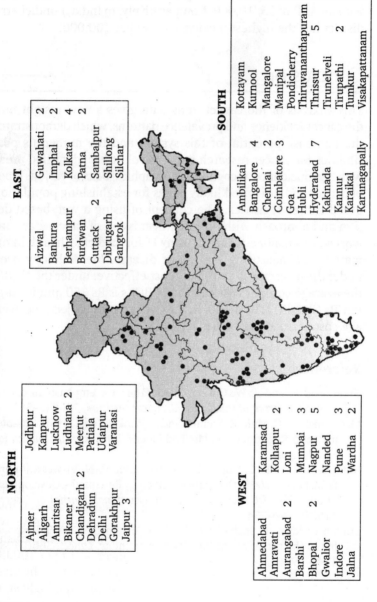

NORTH

Ajmer	Jodhpur
Aligarh	Kanpur
Amritsar	Lucknow
Bikaner	Ludhiana 2
Chandigarh 2	Meerut
Dehradun	Patiala
Delhi	Udaipur
Gorakhpur	Varanasi
Jaipur 3	

EAST

Aizwal	Guwahati 2
Bankura	Imphal 2
Berhampur	Kolkata 4
Burdwan	Patna 2
Cuttack 2	Sambalpur
Dibrugarh	Shillong
Gangtok	Silchar

WEST

Ahmedabad	Karamsad
Amravati	Kolhapur 2
Aurangabad 2	Loni
Barshi	Mumbai 3
Bhopal 2	Nagpur 5
Gwalior	Nanded
Indore	Pune 3
Jalna	Wardha 2

SOUTH

Ambilikai	Kottayam
Bangalore 4	Kurnool
Chennai 2	Mangalore
Coimbatore 3	Manipal
Goa	Pondicherry
Hubli	Thiruvananthapuram
Hyderabad 7	Thrissur 5
Kakinada	Tirunelveli
Kannur	Tirupathi 2
Karaikal	Tumkur
Karunagapally	Visakapattanam

high with an incidence of 26 per 100,000 in Aizwal in Mizoram. Zimbabwe (Africa) has the highest incidence of cervical cancer with an AAR of 55/10,000. Comparatively, in India, Pondicherry district has the highest incidence of 39 per 100,000.

Conclusion

This analysis of the cancer atlas data gives a new insight into the cancer incidence and prevalence patterns, which demonstrates the immense potential of this system and the numerous possibilities for cancer research and control. It has identified areas with high incidence, recognised geographical belts of various types of cancer and discerned likely zones for establishing population based cancer registries. The concept of using a web-based design and approach with online transmission of cancer data has worked as a major advance in using IT for medicine, health informatics and measuring burden of disease. Methodology used under the project was extremely cost-effective: under the NCRP, the average cost per case in urban PBCRs is Rs 350 and in rural PBCRs (Barshi) is Rs 4,100. In the Cancer Atlas Project, the average cost accrued per case is Rs 24.

References

Greenwald P. and J. W. Cullen. 1985. 'The new emphasis in cancer control', *Journal of the National Cancer Institute*, 74: 543–551.

MacLennan R., C. Muir, R. Steinitz and A. Winkler (eds). 1978. 'Chapter in Cancer Registration and Its Techniques', *IARC Scientific Publication No 21*, Lyon.

Nandakumar A., P. C. Gupta, P. Gangadharan, R. N. Visweswara and D. M. Parkin. 2005. 'Geographic Pathology Re-visited—Development of an Atlas of Cancer in India', *International Journal of Cancer*, 116(5): 740–754.

Srinath, Reddy K., B. Shah, C. Varghese and A. Ramadoss. 2005. 'Responding to the threat of chronic diseases in India', *Lancet*, 366(9498): 1744–49.

Health Care Delivery Challenges for Chronic Diseases in India

19

A. VAIDHEESH

Introduction

In the ultimate analysis, any society will be judged by its ability to provide universal health care for its people. This does not merely entail the ability to treat diseases and ailments, but also to prevent their onset by means of suitable systems and measures—President of India on 'Health Care India 2020'.

The Prime Minister of India has also emphasised in his Article, 'Fulfilling India's Promise', 'As a nation, we should be doing more in both health and education. Our total expenditure on health, public and private does not compare favorably with South East Asian countries...and the mix is excessively in favor of private spending'.

As per the estimates, by the year 2050, India will be the third largest economy in the world with the GDP of US dollars 27 trillion, after China and United States (Goldman Sachs 2003). With this statistics, it can be expected that by 2015 the health care expenditure in India will go up to 12 per cent[1] along with 8 per cent increase in the consumer expenditure[2] (Medistate-country profiles National statistical offices, OECD, Eurostat, Euromonitor, Economist Intelligent Unit, ESPICOM 2004). India is still a young country comprising 25 per cent population in the age group of 5–14 years (Census 2001). But it can be seen that the proportion of population, in the age-group of 55 years and above, will increase from 9 per cent to 12 per cent during the year 1991 to 2010 (see Table 19.1). Along with this, the demand of health care for aged population will increase due to improved life expectancy.

Table 19.1 Percentage distribution of target population for health care

Age-group	1991	2001	2010
0–14	36	35	29
15–54	55	55	59
55 and above	9	10	12

Source: Statistical Outline of India 2001–02.

However, in near future, many of the chronic diseases are likely to have severe impact on the quality of life of the aged population of India. The dream of a healthy nation cannot be achieved without serious consideration and necessary actions, such as appropriate awareness of the health care programmes and implementation of screening programmes in public hospitals, rather than managing the conditions of the crippled population.

A health care delivery can only be reframed while changing the approach of the government and the population from the concept of 'Break down health care' to 'Preventive health management'. With the approach, many of the lives and resources can be saved.

The increasing trend towards 'Lifestyle' diseases

Worldwide nearly 5 per cent population (194 million) in the age group 20–79 is estimated to have one or other chronic diseases namely diabetes, arthritis, morbid obesity, anorectal diseases (piles), cardiovascular diseases, gastro-esophageal (GI) reflux diseases, reproductive health diseases (urinary incontinence, menorogia and breast cancer).

In India, obesity, cardiovascular diseases and diabetes are growing enormously. There is a lack of adequate health care infrastructure for the management of the future needs. Many of the developed countries like Japan and the United States do manage such complex situations by adopting the principle of 'preventive health care' rather than 'break down health care management'. For example, in Japan, gastric cancer, suppose to be considered a killer disease two decades ago, is not such a threat anymore. Similarly, in western countries, the menace of breast cancer, which was endemic and life limiting, has been brought down to a significant level, thereby extending the productive longevity. Diabetes and cholesterol are no longer life threatening diseases in many of the developed countries.

A silent disease, diabetes is a cause of many other chronic diseases. Inspite of the latest technology and effective management in India, this ailment may take priority for the coming next 20 years. Presently, India has 35,600,000 diabetes patients (see Figure 19.1). It has been estimated that by 2025 India will be the capital of diabetes with a 73,000,000 adult diabetic population (Projection). Even though it is a simple disease, it requires sustainable social commitment to create awareness and early screening.

India is the second highest country with an estimated 33,000,000 obese population, at a 4.4 per cent growth rate per annum, after USA (53,000,000 obese population) (Frost and Sullivan). Further, after Russians, Indians are more prone to get cardiovascular diseases, with 0.17 per cent increase per annum. Challenges to manage these diseases are daunting and complex. There is a need for proper health care resources (that is, health care centres, health care professionals, drugs and devices) for the management of lifestyle diseases. However, many chronic diseases have a tendency to become chronic because of the lack of early detection and appropriate management programmes. The demand of health care is expected to outstrip supply over the next decade. In this scenario, the future of private medical care providers appears to be very affirmative. Almost 80,000 additional hospital beds will be required per year for the next three to four years to meet the growing health care demands.

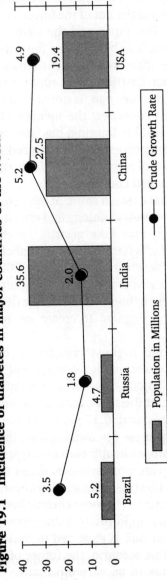

Figure 19.1 Incidence of diabetes in major countries of the world

Source: Frost and Sullivan.

However, public health care system will add only 8,000 beds per year. The available public health care infrastructure in rural and urban areas of the country can be seen in the Table 19.2.

Table 19.2 Public health care infrastructure

Urban	
Tertiarry Medical collages/hospitals	117
ESI and PSU hospitals	1,200
Urban Health Posts	1,500
Rural	
District and Taluk Hospitals	4,400
Community health centres	2,400
Primary health centres	23,000
Sub centres	132,000

Source: ICRA, 2001.

In spite of high incidence of diseases, there is an extremely slow progress in the rates of surgery/intervention. The key contributing factors for the slow progress is the lack of screening programme, trained surgeons/interventional physicians, general practitioners, awareness/ability to 'prescribe' interventional options, ignorance/fear of intervention and lack of health care infrastructure availability like operation theatres and beds. The most important factor, which cannot be ignored, is 'affordability'.

Purchasing power

India's purchasing power is higher than US dollar 20,000, better than China, even though both the countries are facing similar problems. But India has a weak health care infrastructure. From Table 19.3, it can be seen that per thousand population, India has only 1.5 beds, 0.5 physicians, 0.9 nurses, which is quite less as compared to middle and high income countries and world as a whole.

While health care facilities are growing at a fast rate, most of the health needs are taken care of by the private sector. Out of 18,778 numbers of hospitals, 70 per cent belongs to private sector and rest 30 per cent are from public sector. According to Mckinsey CII report, 2001, it can be seen that in total number

Table 19.3   Health infrastructure in India, 2001

	Per 1,000 population		
	Beds	*Physicians*	*Nurses*
India	1.5	0.5	0.9
Middle income countries	4.3	1.8	1.9
High income countries	7.4	1.8	7.5
World Average	3.3	1.5	3.3

Source: Mckinsey CII Report 2001.

of beds in India, the share of government sector is only 38 per cent as compared to the private sector (organised private sector, 23 per cent and unorganised sector, 39 per cent). The proportion of bed is also growing at the rate of 1.1 per cent per annum along with the 3.9 per cent increase in the proportion of doctors (Frost and Sullivan).

India's expenditure on health is Rs. 105 billion, which is 5.2 per cent of the GDP, one of the highest among developing countries. However, its per capita health care expenditure is relatively low at an estimated 24 US dollars (2001). In this scenario, priority should be given for the development of extensive basic health infrastructure, medical education and extensive public hospital system. Further, less than 15 per cent of population is formally covered, through pre-payment, showing the lack of coverage in purchasing power. Whereas, with the low purchasing power, 2/3rd of health care expenditure is out of pocket. Figure 19.2 shows the share of different payers in the total expenditure.

Trends and opportunities in the present scenario

It can be said that in future there will be a rising demand for quality health care. Privatisation has already begun in Indian health care since 1980s. The share of health in the total private expenditure has risen from 3.5 per cent in 1993–94 to 5.3 per cent in 2001–02. However, the tendency of competition with respect to price packages based on low quality practises and mismatch with regulation can be observed. At the same time, an increase in the involvement of private health insurance in the

Figure 19.2   Share of different payers per cent of total expenditure, 2000–01

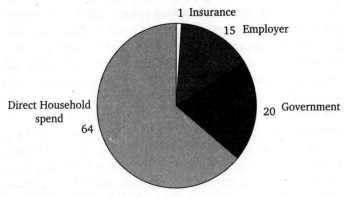

Source: Mckinsey CII Report 2001.

health care market can also be seen and it will be around Rs 1.6 billion by 2010; with the premium of less than US dollar 222 million (MM) (2003). The levels of health insurance is still low due to regulatory and systemic barriers.

There is a huge unmet demand for surgical procedures. In order to train the surgeons, there is an urgent need to forge partnership with educational institutions/industry. Education and awareness programmes need to be conducted for General Physicians (GPs), in order to update their skills in new technology and trends.

India is a patient-pays market with low affordability and reimbursement. There is no need here for the funding models based on USA or UK as the environment is ready for the adoption of heath insurance and innovation in funding models. The best examples of innovative funding models already exist in India. The funding model of Arvind Eye Hospital and Yashaswini scheme for farmers in Karnataka are the models where people of all the strata could have access to health care services.

Summary

Many governments/societies have tackled the challenges faced by the health care system, while having partnership with the industry to put in robust processes to create awareness and drive sustainable mass screening programme. Some of the examples are: mobile breast cancer screening clinics, anorectal screening camps, public forums and web based osteo-arthritis education programme, patient support groups for morbid obesity, diabetes screening camps and education centres, women's health education programmes in the management of uterus and menorogia, etc. In addition, there are three medical education training centres in India to train young health care specialists in emerging technologies like minimal access surgery, infection control seminars, basics surgical skills, arthritis management, etc. However, as a commercial organisation, the health care industry has its own limitations in implementing large-scale awareness, screening camps and education programmes for health care professionals/patients. Hence, it is important that policy makers in the government work with the industry to update the educational curriculum of health care professionals and prioritise the diseases and states that need to be tackled immediately.

Notes

1. based on ESPICOM 2002–12 forecast.
2. based on Economic Intelligence Unit (EIU) 2003–08 forecast.

References

Ashok Alexander *et al.* 2002. *Health care in India: The Road Ahead*, CII and Mekinsey and Company. Available online at http://www.aippg.net/forum/viewtopic.php?t=52214 (accessed on 16 October 2007).

Census of India 2001. Available online at http://www.censusindia.net/

Dominic Wilson and Reopa Purushottaman. 2003. 'Dreaming with BRICs: the Path to 2050', Global Economics Paper No. 99, Goldman Sachs Group Inc. Available online at http://www2.goldmansachs.com/insight/research/reports/99.pdf (accessed on 16 October 2007).

Economic Intelligence Unit (EIU), a division of *The Economist* working in the area of global business.

Frost and Sullivan, Diabetes Drug Delivery Methods—Market and Technologies, http://www.marketresearch.com/search/results. asp?SID=69717311-376131964-307010627&qtype=2&publisher =Frost+%26+Sullivan&query=diabetes&categoryid=1594&regi onid=1407&mcats=Health care

Frost and Sullivan, World Emerging Anti-Obesity Prescription Drug Markets. Available online at http://www.marketresearch.com/ search/results.asp?SID=69717311-376131964-307010627&qty pe=2&publisher=Frost+%26+Sullivan&query=diabetes&categ oryid=1594&regionid=1407&mcats=Health care (accessed on 16 October 2007).

ICRA. 2001. Report on Health care Indicators. Available online at www.buyusa.gov/virginia/indiahealth care.pdf (accessed on 16 October 2007).

Medistat Outlook ESPICOM Report January 2004.

Rajat K. Gupta. 2005. 'India's Economic Agenda: An Interview with Manmohan Singh', *The McKinsey Quarterly-Special Edition: Fulfilling India's promise.* Available online at http://www.mckinseyquarterly. com/article_page.aspx?ar=1674&l2=19&l3=67 (accessed on 16 October 2007).

Statistical Outline of India 2001–02. Department of Economics and Statistics, Tata Services, Mumbai.

About the Editors and Contributors

Editors

K.V. Ramani was Chairman of the Centre for Management of Health Services, Public Systems Group, Indian Institute of Management, Ahmedabad (IIMA) (2004–2007), obtained his Ph.D degree in Operations Research from Cornell University, USA in 1977. He is also a Visiting Professor at the Leeds University Business School, UK. Dr Ramani has served as a member on the IIMA Board of Governors.

Dr Ramani has published extensively in international refereed journals such as Journal of Health Organization and Management, Interfaces, Naval Research Logistics, Journal of Strategic Information Systems, Computers & Education, Simulation among others. He has been a consultant to the Commonwealth Secretariat, World Bank, European Commission, DfID, and a number of hospitals in India and abroad.

His teaching and research interests are in hospital logistics management, urban health and HIV/AIDS. Some of his ongoing research projects are on management capacity assessment for RCH Program; health policy in India, China, and Vietnam; managing urban health; social obligations for Cancer care; case studies on safe motherhood; managerial challenges in HIV/AIDS, and corruption in health systems, University of Leeds.

Dileep Mavalankar is Associate Professor, Public Systems Group, IIMA, and has a doctorate in public health from Johns Hopkins University, USA and a doctorate in medicine from Gujarat University. He has worked in various research and academic institutions including National Institute of Health in Bethesda, USA, NHL Medical College, Ahmedabad and Columbia University, USA. Dr Mavalankar has authored over

20 publications on public health and health management topics. He has been consultant/adviser of numerous organisations and governments, including the Mother Care Project, USA, the World Health Organization, Geneva, Philippines and China, the Aga Khan Foundation among others. He also has worked with several NGOs in India. He has been on editorial boards of some public health journals.

His present work includes improving management of emergency obstetric care in rural hospitals; strengthening reproductive health programme management; improving the quality of care in family welfare; health policy analysis and implications; collaboration of NGO and the government in health programmes and management of the service sector and quality of services.

Dipti Govil is currently associated with Centre for Management of Health Services, Indian Institute of Management, Ahmedabad and working on health policy process in India. She holds a Ph.D. and masters degree in Population Studies from International Institute of Population Sciences, Mumbai. Her specific interests include community and women's health, population and development, health system and quality of care. She has also worked on blood banking services in India.

Contributors

Sonia Andrews is currently pursuing her doctoral degree at University of Perth, Australia. She holds a Masters degree in economics and public health. Her interests include the role of private health sector and the economic impact of communicable diseases.

Urvashi Chandra has been working in the development sector for about seven years particularly in the area of public health. She has worked for international organizations such as BBC World Service Trust, Johns Hopkins University Centre for Communications Programs, UNICEF, and Delegation of the European Commission in India and the German Agency for Technical Cooperation. Her areas of specialization include reproductive & child health, maternal & child health, health sector reforms and HIV/AIDS. She obtained her doctoral degree in Sociology from Jawaharlal Nehru University, Delhi in 2003.

Joe Curian is presently President, Association of Hospitals and the chief spokesperson; member, Confederation of Indian Industry (CII) National Committee on Healthcare, co-chairman, Federation of Indian Chambers of Commerce and Industry (FICCI) National Committee on Healthcare and President elect of the Indian Healthcare Federation.

He is currently involved with the turnaround of S L Raheja Hospital—a 250 bed capacity hospital. He contributes regularly to important publications on healthcare and has presented a number of papers both in India and abroad.

Joe Curian holds a Masters in Management Studies (MMS) and a post-graduate degree from the prestigious Defence Services Staff College. He participated in both the India-Pakistan wars and was decorated for gallantry on both the occasions.

Having sought premature retirement from the Army, he joined as CEO of various hospitals including Apollo Hospitals, Chennai and Delhi. The former received ISO 9000 certification under him. Later, he took over as CEO, P D Hinduja National Hospital & Medical Research Centre, Mumbai.

Michael Friedman is the Associate Director, South India for CDC/Global AIDS Program—India and the senior physician for the US Government in India. He holds the rank of Commander in the US Public Health Services. Prior to coming to India, he has had extensive experience working as an internist and pediatrician and has led CDC efforts related to diabetes, obesity, asthma and air pollution. As part of his previous responsibilities, he has had the opportunity to work closely with the private health care industry on issues of continuous quality improvement and standards of care. He is currently working on incorporating some of these strategies into the current efforts in India to address HIV and AIDS.

Nancy Gerein holds a Ph.D in Health Care Epidemiology from the London School of Hygiene and Tropical Medicine and a M.Sc in Health Policy and Planning from the University of British Columbia in Canada. She has worked in India as a nursing instructor, in Cameroon in community health and in Indonesia as a health planner. For 10 years she was a health advisor for the Canadian International Development Agency, responsible for the planning, management and evaluation of health projects in Africa and Asia. More recently, she was the director of a CIDA-funded programme of support to the health and population sector in Bangladesh. Since joining the Nuffield Institute in 1999, she manages the research programme in reproductive health, and does teaching and consultancy in the areas of reproductive health, health systems development and monitoring and evaluation.

Meenakshi Datta Ghosh belongs to the Indian Administrative Service and is presently Secretary, Ministry of Panchayati Raj, and Government of India. She was responsible for formulating the National Population Policy, 2000. Her special interests are in the areas of decentralization of health care and convergence of service delivery.

She is a Ph.D. candidate at the University of Pittsburgh, USA, in the field of Public Policy Research and Analysis. She has a Masters in Public Policy, Kennedy School of Government, Harvard University; a Masters in Sociology, Delhi School of Economics Delhi University as well as Diplomas in French and Russian. Ms Ghosh has held several positions of responsibility in development administration. She has motivated the updating of standards and specifications of contraceptives and instrumentation used in the national family welfare programme.

Andrew Green is Professor of International Health Planning and Head of the Nuffield Centre for International Health and Development, a WHO Collaborating Centre, at the University of Leeds, UK. He studied politics and economics as a first degree, then Development Economics at the Masters level and was awarded a Ph.D for work focusing on health planning and policy. In the late 1970s, he set up and headed the National Health Planning Unit for the Government of Swaziland and following this, worked in the UK as a planner focusing on primary care. His current research focuses on health systems and health policy processes. He is currently a member of the WHO Global Advisory Group on Nursing and Midwifery. His book *An Introduction to Health Planning for Developing Health Systems* (OUP, 2007) is a widely used text.

Stephen Jan is a senior health economist at the George Institute for International Health at Sydney, Australia. Earlier he was with the Health Policy Unit of the London School of Hygiene and Tropical Medicine (London). His research interests include institutional economics, regulator and financing issues and role of NGOs in developing countries.

Ardi Kaptiningsih is Regional Adviser, Reproductive Health and Research, Family and Community Health Department, WHO/SEARO. She graduated from the Faculty of Medicine, University of Padjadjaran, Bandung, Indonesia in 1978 and obtained her Masters degree in Nutrition and Maternal and Child Health, School of Public Health, University of North Carolina at Chapel Hill, NC, USA in 1986.

Sweta Mehandiratta is Research Associate at the Indian Institute of Management, Ahmedabad. She is working on urban health and her specific interests are in the area of occupational health and community health. Ms Mehandiratta has worked as a health coordinator with Self Employed Women's Association (SEWA) and as a dietician at Shri Krishna Hospital and Pramukh Swami Medical College, Karamsad. She holds a Masters in Food & Nutrition, Sardar Patel University.

V.R. Muraleedharan is Professor of Economics in the Department of Humanities and Social Sciences, Indian Institute of Technology, Madras. His current research work spans issues on financing, human resources, regulation and new public management approaches to health care in India. He has carried out historical research in health care in colonial South India.

A. Nandakumar is Deputy Director General (Senior Grade), Indian Council of Medical Research (ICMR) as well as office-in-charge. He has completed his MBBS and MD (Pathology) from

Bangalore Medical College, Bangalore University in 1981. He completed Masters in Public Health (Epidemiology) in 1987–89 from School of Public Health and Community Medicine, University of Washington, Seattle, USA. He has received Fellowship of International Union against Cancer and International Agency for Research on Cancer. He has published over 50 books and papers in national and international journals.

Amit Patel is currently working as a Research Associate at the Indian Institute of Management, Ahmedabad. He is working on urban health and his specific interest is in the area of healthcare infrastructure planning. He has also worked on design of public hospitals. He holds a Masters in Urban and Regional Planning from the Center for Environmental Planning & Technology (CEPT) and Bachelors in Architecture, M.S. University of Baroda.

Keerti Bhusan Pradhan is a post-graduate in Health Management from Tata Institute of Social Sciences (TISS), Mumbai and is working in the health sector for last 15 years. Presently he is working with LAICO-Aravind Eye Care System as a Management faculty and head of Capacity Building Initiative. He has undergone additional training at CDC-Atlanta on Management of International Public Health.

His expertise has been in the field of public health management, community ophthalmology and eye care management. As a consultant he is providing support to many organizations in India and outside India.

He also provides training to professionals in health management from developing countries. He also helps non-eye care NGOs in having eye care services integrated to their health and development work for their service population. His main focus has been on capacity building of organizations with a focus on systems, procedures, human resources, policies and strategies.

Bhuvaneswari R. is currently a freelance researcher in Mumbai. She holds a Masters degree in economics and has considerable experience in conducting studies on costing public health interventions, with particular reference to preventive strategies against HIV/AIDS and tuberculosis.

Aruna Rabel is the Medical Administration Manager of Durdans Hospital, Colombo, which is one of the major private hospitals in Sri Lanka. He has been appointed as a Member of the Private Health Institutions Regulatory Council in Sri Lanka in the year 2006. He obtained his MBBS in 1991 and Masters Degree in Medical Administration from the Post Graduate Institute of Medicine, University of Colombo in 2003.

G.N.V. Ramana is a public health physician with expertise in large scale social sector program management and operations research in developing countries. Since 1998 he is working as a Senior Public Health Specialist with the World Bank at New Delhi. He has obtained Masters in Community Health, Certificate in Applied Nutrition, Bachelor in Medicine and Surgery.

He is the first to be awarded honours by Osmania University under the Masters Program in Community Medicine, 1989. He also received awards for best overall and statistical papers at the State level annual public health conferences as well as the Spot and performance awards at the World Bank. He has published two papers in international journals, written nine analytical reports and published three other papers as a lead author and four papers as a co-author.

S.R. Rao joined the Indian Administrative Service in the year 1978 and is presently working as Principal Secretary, Urban Development and Urban Housing Department, Government of Gujarat, India. He has extensively worked in developmental infrastructure sector, field of rural development, industry, urban development, port and nuclear energy. He received his Masters degrees in Applied Sociology from Andhra University and Rural Development from University of East Anglia, UK.

He received the National Science Foundation Award for Public Health in 1996, All India Management Association Award for Excellence in Public Service in 1997, United Nations Habitat Award for Best Practices in 1997 Eisenhower Fellow in the year 1998, and was conferred the Padma Shri by the Government of India in 1998.

Jeffrey D. Sachs is the Director of The Earth Institute, Quetelet Professor of Sustainable Development, and Professor of Health Policy and Management at Columbia University. From 2002 to 2006, he was Director of the UN Millennium Project and Special Advisor to United Nations Secretary-General Kofi Annan on the Millennium Development Goals, the internationally agreed goals to reduce extreme poverty, disease, and hunger by the year 2015. For more than 20 years, Professor Sachs has been at the forefront of the challenges of economic development, poverty alleviation, and enlightened globalization, promoting policies to help all parts of the world to benefit from expanding economic opportunities and well-being. He is also one of the leading voices for combining economic development with environmental sustainability, and as Director of the Earth Institute leads large-scale efforts to promote the mitigation of human-induced climate change. He was named among the 100 most influential leaders in the world by *Time Magazine* in 2004 and 2005, and is the recipient of the Sargent Shriver Award for Equal Justice, 2005. He is author of many scholarly articles and books, including New York Times bestseller *The End of Poverty* (Penguin, 2005). He has received many honorary degrees, most recently from Trinity College Dublin, the College of the Atlantic, Southern Methodist University, Simon Fraser University and McGill University. A native of Detroit, Michigan, Sachs received his B.A., M.A., and Ph.D. degrees at Harvard University.

Rajeev Sadanandan is a research student at Jawaharlal Nehru University, New Delhi. Formerly he was health secretary, Kerala and has worked with UNAIDS India country office. He played a pivotal role in developing the Project Implementation Plan for the third phase of the National AIDS Control Programme.

Sangeeta Singh, a social scientist by training has been involved in the field of social development since the past 10 years. Presently working as a consultant, she holds a post-graduate degree from the Tata Institute of Social Sciences, Mumbai and M.Phil. in public health from Jawaharlal Nehru University, Delhi. She began her work in the field of public health from *Seva Mandir,*

Udaipur a non-government organisation working with tribal and poor rural communities in Udaipur and surrounding districts. Her interest areas are research on health rights, participation of communities and accountability.

H. Sudarshan is an MBBS from Bangalore Medical College, Adjunct Professor, Indira Gandhi National Open University and Honorary Fellow of the Association of Rural Surgeons of India. Besides, he has been the member in many state and national bodies like National Literacy Mission, Steering group of Planning Commission, Working Group of Ninth Five Year Plan, Steering Committee on Health for Tenth Five Year plan, Confederation of Indian Industry (CII) among others.

Presently he is working as a Vigilance Director, Karnataka Lokayukta (Health, Education & Social Welfare), Government of Karnataka, India.

He is also a member of national and state level organisations like the National Commission on Population, State Wildlife Advisory Board, Karnataka State Literacy Mission Authority, Indira Gandhi National Open University, National Nutrition Mission and so on. He has received many awards and medals including Right Livelihood Award (Alternate Nobel Prize), Sweden in 1994 and the Padmashree in 2000.

A. Vaidheesh is presently working as executive Vice-President—Medical devices, India. He has been member of the leadership team, actively involving in corporate initiatives namely Signature of Quality and process excellence. He has also been responsible for dramatically accelerating the business growth of a new franchise through a well thought out roadmap and strategic plan and also for supply chain and strategic marketing and process excellence for the entire organization.

He has been the member of Asia-Pacific strategy council and leader of Global Umbrella task force for 'Direct to consumer' initiative. Base: Mumbai and is reporting to President. He has obtained masters degree in Management.

Index

Indian Institute of Management, Ahmedabad, India
Centre for Management of Health Services (CMHS)

Policy, Planning, Evaluation
Macro Economic Analysis
Health Sector Reforms
District Health System
Public Health System
Private Healthcare
Urban Healthcare
Public-Private Partnerships
National Programmes
(RCH, HIV/AIDS, Cancer...)
Allied Sectors (Nutrition, Pharma...)

Building Health Systems
Operations Research
IT applications
Healthcare Logistics
Service Quality Improvements
Human Resources Management
Financial Management
Health Insurance
Management Information Systems
Linkages with Pharma, Med Equip,...

Research Projects

State/District Health Officers
Hospital Managers and Administrators
Nursing Managers and Administrators
NGOs

Capacity Building

Dissemination

Institution Building

Seminars
Workshops
Conferences

Synergy with other institutions